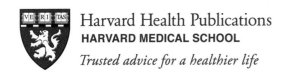

Harvard Health Publications
HARVARD MEDICAL SCHOOL

Trusted advice for a healthier life

D1239962

Dear Reader,

How do you feel when you wake up in the morning? Are you refreshed and ready to go, or groggy and grumpy? For many people, the second scenario is all too common. About 70 million Americans of all ages suffer from chronic sleep problems, according to the Centers for Disease Control and Prevention. Insomnia—trouble falling or staying asleep—is the most common complaint, but other chronic disorders, including sleep apnea, restless legs syndrome, or narcolepsy, can also contribute to a shut-eye shortfall. And some people simply stay up too late—usually because they're watching late-night TV, according to a national time-use survey of more than 21,000 adults. Logging long hours on the computer is another common cause of sleep loss.

Regardless of the reason, as many as one in three Americans sleeps less than six hours a night—a trend that can have serious personal and public health consequences. According to a 2015 consensus statement from the American Academy of Sleep Medicine and the Sleep Research Society, all adults should get seven or more hours of sleep a night.

Insufficient sleep can make you too tired to work efficiently, to exercise, or to eat healthfully. Over time, sleep deprivation increases the risk for a number of chronic health problems, including obesity, diabetes, high blood pressure, and heart disease. What's more, one in 24 of American drivers admitted to falling asleep while driving at least once in the previous month, according to a government report. Some estimates suggest drowsy driving accounts for up to a quarter of fatal highway crashes.

Even though many people acknowledge that sleep is important, few seek treatment for their sleep problems. But you needn't fumble about in a fog of fatigue. This report features the latest studies on cognitive behavioral therapy, a drug-free technique to treat insomnia; information on how to safely use prescription sleep medications; and ways to recognized uncommon sleep disorders, such as narcolepsy and nocturnal eating syndrome. You'll also learn about the growing use of a portable home test to detect sleep apnea, an underrecognized yet life-threatening sleep disorder. Most importantly, we include reliable, time-tested remedies to help you get the sleep you need for optimal health, safety, and well-being.

Sincerely,

Lawrence Epstein, M.D.
Medical Editor

Sleep mechanics

For centuries, scientists scrutinized minute aspects of human activity, but showed little interest in the time that people spent in sleep. Sleep seemed inaccessible to medical probing—a subject best suited to poets and dream interpreters who could conjure meaning out of the void. It was thought to be no more than a natural reaction to the darkness and silence of night, when the brain could no longer react to the sensory stimulation of the day. Scientists believed the brain was simply "turned off" and remained unchanged throughout the night.

All that changed in the 1930s, when researchers found they could place sensitive electrodes on the scalp and record the signals produced by electrical activity in the brain to create electroencephalograms, or EEGs. When this technique revealed lively brain activity even in sleeping subjects, scientists realized that sleep did not represent a void, but was in fact a dynamic time, incorporating different stages with markedly different patterns of brain waves. Further study revealed that it is a period when the brain consolidates memories and cleans out toxins, when growth and development occur, and when the immune system surveys the body for potential problems.

Far from being a luxury, sleep is now known to be essential, required for health and optimal functioning. Sleep deprivation can be used as a form of torture. Yet many of us continue to get inadequate sleep—either because we deliberately deprive ourselves of sleep or because we seem unable to get a good night's rest.

This report will delve into the many steps you can take to restore sleep quality. But first, it may help to review the different stages of sleep and what scientists

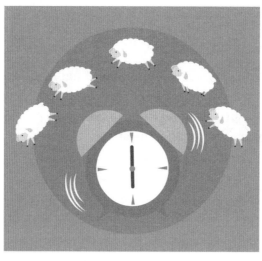

Thinkstock

call "sleep architecture," meaning the patterns of alternating sleep stages you pass through during the night.

Quiet (non-REM) sleep

Scientists divide sleep into two major types: REM (rapid eye movement) sleep or dreaming sleep, and non-REM or quiet sleep. Surprisingly, they are as different from each other as either is from waking.

Sleep specialists have called non-REM sleep "an idling brain in a movable body." During this phase, thinking and most bodily functions slow down, but movement can still occur, and a person often shifts position while sinking into deeper stages of sleep.

To an extent, the idea of "dropping" into sleep parallels changes in brain-wave patterns at the onset of non-REM sleep. When you are awake, billions of brain cells receive and analyze sensory information and coordinate behavior by sending electrical impulses to one another. If you're fully awake, an EEG records a messy, irregular scribble of activity. Once your eyes are closed and your brain no longer receives visual input, brain waves settle into a steady and rhythmic pattern of about 10 cycles per second. This is the alpha-wave pattern, characteristic of calm, relaxed wakefulness (see Figure 1, page 3).

The transition to quiet sleep is a quick one that might be likened to flipping a switch—that is, you are either awake (switch on) or asleep (switch off). Some brain centers and pathways stimulate the entire brain to wakefulness; others promote falling asleep. One brain chemical, hypocretin (also called orexin), seems to play an important role in regulating when the flip between states occurs and keeping you in the new state. Interestingly, people with a condition called narcolepsy often lack hypocretin, and as a result they frequently flip back and forth between sleep and wakefulness, suddenly falling asleep during the day or at other inappropriate times for short bouts known as "sleep attacks."

Unless something disturbs the process, you proceed smoothly through the three stages of quiet sleep.

Stage N1

In making the transition from wakefulness into light sleep, you spend about five minutes in stage N1 sleep. On the EEG, the predominant brain waves slow to four to seven cycles per second, a pattern called theta waves (see Figure 1, at right). Body temperature begins to drop, muscles relax, and eyes often move slowly from side to side. People in stage N1 sleep lose awareness of their surroundings, but they are easily jarred awake. However, not everyone experiences stage N1 sleep in the same way: if awakened, one person might recall being drowsy, while another might describe having been asleep.

Stage N2

This first stage of true sleep lasts 10 to 25 minutes. Your eyes are still, and your heart rate and breathing are slower than when awake. Your brain's electrical activity is irregular. Large, slow waves intermingle with brief bursts of activity called sleep spindles, when brain waves speed up for roughly half a second or longer. Scientists believe that when spindles occur, the brain disconnects from outside sensory input and begins the process of memory consolidation (which involves organizing memories for long-term storage). The EEG tracings also show a pattern called a K-complex, which scientists think represents a sort of built-in vigilance system that keeps you poised to awaken if necessary. K-complexes can also be provoked by certain sounds or other external or internal stimuli. Whisper someone's name during stage N2 sleep, and a K-complex will appear on the EEG. You spend about half the night in stage N2 sleep.

Stage N3 (deep sleep, or slow-wave sleep)

Eventually, large, slow brain waves called delta waves become a major feature on the EEG, and you enter deep sleep. Breathing becomes more regular. Blood pressure falls, and the pulse slows to about 20% to 30% below the waking rate. The brain is less responsive to external stimuli, making it difficult to wake the sleeper.

Deep sleep seems to be a time for your body to renew and repair itself. Blood flow is directed less toward your brain, which cools measurably. At the beginning of this stage, the pituitary gland releases a pulse of growth hormone that stimulates tissue growth and muscle repair. Researchers have also detected increased blood levels of substances that activate your immune system, raising the possibility that deep sleep helps the body defend itself against infection.

Figure 1: EEG brain wave patterns during sleep

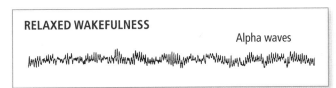

RELAXED WAKEFULNESS
Alpha waves

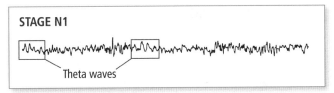

STAGE N1
Theta waves

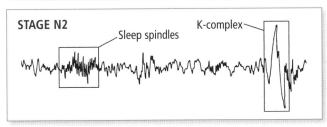

STAGE N2
Sleep spindles
K-complex

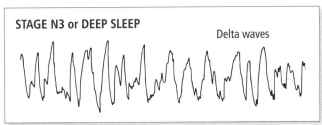

STAGE N3 or DEEP SLEEP
Delta waves

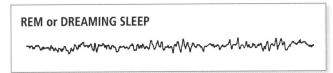

REM or DREAMING SLEEP

Brain waves change dramatically during the different stages of sleep.

Normally, young people spend about 20% of their sleep time in stretches of deep sleep lasting up to half an hour, but deep sleep is nearly absent in most people over age 65 (see "The later years," page 9). When you sleep after a period of sleep deprivation, you pass quickly through the lighter sleep stages into the deeper stages and spend a greater proportion of sleep time there. This suggests that deep sleep plays a large part in restoring alertness and fills an essential role in a person's optimal functioning.

Dreaming (REM) sleep

Dreaming occurs during REM sleep, which has been described as an "active brain in a paralyzed body." Your brain races, thinking and dreaming, as your eyes dart back and forth rapidly behind closed lids. Your body temperature rises. Your blood pressure increases, and your heart rate and breathing speed up to daytime levels. The sympathetic nervous system, which creates the fight-or-flight response, is twice as active as when you're awake. Despite all this activity, your body hardly moves, except for intermittent twitches; muscles not needed for breathing or eye movement are quiet.

Just as deep sleep restores your body, scientists believe that REM or dreaming sleep restores your mind, perhaps in part by helping clear out irrelevant information. Studies of students' ability to solve a complex puzzle involving abstract shapes suggest the brain processes information overnight; students who got a good night's sleep after seeing the puzzle fared much better than those asked to solve the puzzle immediately. Earlier studies found that REM sleep facilitates learning and memory. People tested to measure how well they had learned a new task improved their scores after a night's sleep. If they were subjected to periodic awakenings that prevented them from having REM sleep, the improvements were lost. By contrast, if they were awakened an equal number of times from deep sleep, the improvements in the scores were unaf-

Why do we dream?

For centuries, dreams have captivated scholars and everyday people alike, who wonder if the seemingly random thoughts, images, and sensations that occur during sleep hold any special meaning or purpose. What, if anything, can you read into a dream in which you arrive at your senior prom in overalls, or one where you're chased through the streets of Paris by a giant turtle? Though there have been many theories over the years, the meaning of dreams is still a matter of debate.

One famous work on the subject, Sigmund Freud's *The Interpretation of Dreams*, published in 1899, explored why people dream and what dreams reveal about their psychological lives. Freud believed that dreams reveal hidden conflicts, desires, and fears, albeit in disguised form. Other psychoanalytic thinkers later elaborated on and refined his ideas, suggesting that dreams help people organize their thoughts as well as consolidate and reinforce their long-term memories.

The technological advances that enabled EEG recordings during sleep gave rise to alternate theories, like the "activation synthesis hypothesis," which holds that dreams are triggered by random electrical impulses generated during REM sleep. The dream is the brain's attempt to make sense and a cohesive story out of the randomly generated memories. In this theory, the meaning of the dreams is not significant, and the evidence is that we remember so few of them. (In fact, whether or not you can remember a dream seems to depend mainly on one factor—how close to the dreaming period you wake up. However, people can train themselves to remember dreams better by writing them down when they wake up.)

In yet another interpretation, evolutionary psychologists point to the well-documented realistic aspects of dreams as evidence that dreams serve a purpose. The "threat simulation theory" suggests that dreams in which people react to a threatening event (like being attacked by a tiger) help them rehearse for danger in real life. This mental practice during sleep, they postulate, could offer a survival advantage.

In fact, dreaming probably serves multiple functions, but at the very least it seems to be involved in learning and memory. Newborns and young children, who are in a period of intense learning, spend far more time in REM sleep than adults. But REM is not solely responsible for memory consolidation. Studies at Harvard's Beth Israel Deaconess Medical Center have found that both REM and non-REM sleep play a role. Spatial memory, such as remembering where things are located, is enhanced by non-REM sleep, while memories with emotional content are enhanced by REM sleep.

We may not know exactly what function dreaming serves, but the fact that other species such as dogs dream, too, suggests that it plays a fundamental biological role. Life would certainly be less interesting without it.

fected. These findings may help explain why students who stay up all night cramming for an examination generally retain less information than classmates who get some sleep.

About three to five times a night, or about every 90 minutes, you enter REM sleep. The first such episode usually lasts for only a few minutes, but REM time increases progressively over the course of the night. The final period of REM sleep may last a half-hour. If you're deprived of REM sleep and then allowed a subsequent night of undisturbed sleep, you will enter this stage earlier and spend a higher proportion of sleep time in it—a phenomenon called REM rebound.

Sleep architecture

During the night, a normal sleeper moves between different sleep stages in a fairly predictable pattern, alternating between REM and non-REM sleep. When these stages are charted on a diagram, called a hypnogram (see Figure 2, below), the different levels resemble a drawing of a city skyline. Sleep experts call this pattern sleep architecture.

In a young adult, normal sleep architecture usually consists of four or five alternating non-REM and REM periods. Most deep sleep occurs in the first half of the night. As the night progresses, periods of REM sleep get longer and alternate with stage N2 sleep. Later in life, the sleep skyline will change, with less stage N3 sleep, more stage N1 sleep, and more awakenings.

Control of many of the features of sleep architecture resides in the brainstem, the area that also controls breathing, blood pressure, and heartbeat. Fluctuating activity in the nerve cells and the chemical messengers they produce seem to coordinate the timing of wakefulness, arousal, and the 90-minute changeover that occurs between REM and non-REM sleep.

Several neurotransmitters (brain chemicals that neurons release to communicate with adjacent cells) play a role in arousal. Adenosine and gamma-aminobutyric acid (GABA) are believed to promote sleep. Acetylcholine regulates REM sleep. Norepinephrine, epinephrine, dopamine, and hypocretin stimulate wakefulness. Individuals vary greatly in their natural levels of neurotransmitters and in their sensitivity to these chemicals. Many sleep medications are designed to mimic or counteract their effects.

Your internal clock

Certain brain structures and chemicals produce the states of sleeping and waking. For instance, a pacemaker-like mechanism in the brain regulates circadian rhythms. ("Circadian" means "about a day.") This internal clock, which gradually becomes established during the first months of life, controls the daily ups and downs of biological patterns, including body temperature, blood pressure, and the release of hormones.

Circadian rhythms make people's desire for sleep strongest between midnight and dawn, and to a lesser extent in midafternoon. In one study, researchers instructed a group of people to try to stay awake for 24 hours. Not surprisingly, many slipped into naps despite their best efforts not to. When the investigators plotted the times when unplanned naps occurred, they found peaks between 2 a.m. and 4 a.m. and between 2 p.m. and 3 p.m.

Most Americans sleep during the night as dictated by their circadian rhythms, although many who work on weekdays nap in the afternoon on the weekends. In societies where taking a siesta is the norm, people can respond to their bodies' daily dips in alertness with a one- to two-hour afternoon nap during the workday and a correspondingly shorter sleep at night.

Figure 2: Sleep architecture

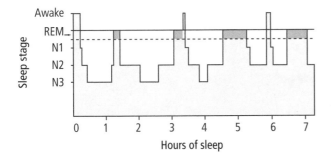

When experts chart sleep stages on a hypnogram, the different levels resemble a drawing of a city skyline. This pattern is known as sleep architecture. The hypnogram above shows a typical night's sleep of a healthy young adult.

In the 1970s, studies in rats identified a brain structure called the suprachiasmatic nucleus as the location of the internal clock. This cluster of cells is part of the hypothalamus, the brain center that regulates appetite and other biological states (see Figure 3, below). When this tiny area was damaged, the sleep/wake rhythm disappeared and the rats no longer slept on a normal schedule. Although the clock is largely self-regulating, its location allows it to respond to several types of external cues to keep it set at 24 hours. Scientists call these cues "zeitgebers," a German word meaning "time givers."

Light. Light striking your eyes is the most influential zeitgeber. When researchers invited volunteers into the laboratory and exposed them to light at intervals that were at odds with the outside world, the participants unconsciously reset their biological clocks to match the new light input. Exposure to light at the right time helps keep the circadian clock on the correct time schedule. However, exposure at the wrong time can shift sleep and wakefulness to undesired times. The circadian rhythm disturbances and sleep problems that affect up to 90% of blind people demonstrate the importance of light to sleep/wake patterns.

Time. As a person reads clocks, follows work and train schedules, and demands that the body remain alert for certain tasks and social events, there is cognitive pressure to stay on schedule.

Melatonin. Cells in the suprachiasmatic nucleus contain receptors for melatonin, a hormone produced in a predictable daily rhythm by the pineal gland, which is located deep in the brain between the two hemispheres. Levels of melatonin begin climbing after dark and ebb after dawn. The hormone induces drowsiness, and scientists believe its daily light-sensitive cycles help keep the sleep/wake cycle on track. ▼

Figure 3: The sleep/wake control center

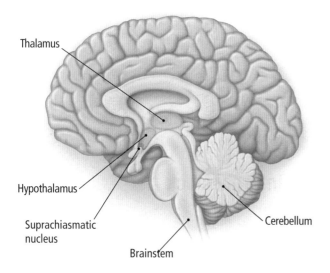

Thalamus

Hypothalamus

Suprachiasmatic nucleus

Brainstem

Cerebellum

The pacemaker-like mechanism in your brain that regulates the circadian rhythm of sleeping and waking is thought to be located in the suprachiasmatic nucleus. This cluster of cells is part of the hypothalamus, the brain center that regulates appetite, body temperature, and other biological states.

Sleep throughout life

To a certain extent, heredity determines how people sleep throughout their lives. Identical twins, for example, have much more similar sleep patterns than nonidentical twins or other sibling pairs. Differences in sleeping and waking seem to be inborn, although the genetic underpinnings aren't fully understood. Scientists have discovered two genetic mutations relating to sleep duration (see "A gene that affects circadian rhythms," page 9). Nevertheless, many factors can affect how a person sleeps. Aging is the most important influence on basic sleep rhythms—from age 20 on, it takes progressively longer to fall asleep. You sleep less each night, stages N1 and N2 sleep increase, deep sleep and REM decrease, and you awaken more often during the night (see Table 1, page 8).

Childhood

For an adult to sleep like a baby is not only unrealistic but also undesirable. A newborn may sleep eight times a day, accumulating 18 hours of sleep and spending about half of it in REM sleep. REM periods occur often, usually less than an hour apart.

At about the age of 4 weeks, a newborn's sleep periods get longer. By 6 months, infants spend longer and more regular periods in non-REM sleep; most begin sleeping through the night and taking naps in the morning and afternoon. During the preschool years, daytime naps gradually shorten, until by age 6 most children are awake all day and sleep for about 10 hours a night.

Between age 7 and puberty, nocturnal melatonin production is at its lifetime peak,

Thinkstock

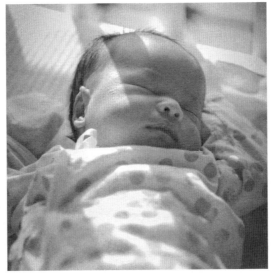

A newborn may sleep 18 hours a day, spending about half of it in REM sleep (dreaming sleep). By 6 months, infants spend more time in non-REM sleep.

and sleep at this age is deep and restorative. At this age, if a child is sleepy during the day, parents should be concerned.

Adolescence

Teenagers need about an hour more sleep each night than they did as young children. But most of them actually sleep an hour or so less. Many factors contribute to the problem, such as drinking caffeinated beverages or staying up too late doing homework or texting friends. But teens' natural sleep/wake cycles also begin to shift up to two hours later once they reach puberty. That means they may not be sleepy until well after their bedtime the night before and may have difficulty waking up early enough to get to school on time.

Research shows that early high school start times contribute to sleep deprivation among teens, which can lead to mood swings, behavioral problems, and difficulties with concentration and learning. Adolescents who get enough sleep are less likely to be overweight, suffer from depression, or be involved in a car accident. They're also more likely to have better grades and a higher quality of life. In response to this evidence, the American Academy of Pediat-

Table 1: Sleep changes during adulthood

As people age, it takes longer to fall asleep, a phenomenon called increased sleep latency. And sleep efficiency—the percentage of time spent asleep while in bed—decreases as well.

	AGE 20	AGE 40	AGE 60	AGE 70	AGE 80
Time to fall asleep	16 minutes	17 minutes	18 minutes	18.5 minutes	19 minutes
Total sleep time	7.5 hours	7 hours	6.2 hours	6 hours	5.8 hours
Time in stage N2 sleep	47%	51%	53%	55%	57%
Time in stage N3 sleep	20%	15%	10%	9%	7.5%
Time in REM sleep	22%	21%	20%	19%	17%
Time asleep while in bed	95%	88%	84%	82%	79%

Source: Sleep, Nov. 1, 2004, pp. 1255–73.

rics issued a policy statement in 2014 recommending that middle and high schools delay start times to 8:30 a.m. or later.

Adulthood

During young adulthood, sleep patterns usually seem stable but in fact are slowly evolving. Between age 20 and age 30, the amount of deep sleep drops by about half, and nighttime awakenings double. By age 40, deep sleep is markedly reduced.

Women's reproductive cycles can greatly influence sleep. During the first trimester of pregnancy, many women are sleepy all the time and may log an extra two hours a night if their schedules permit. As pregnancy continues, hormonal and anatomical changes make sound, restful sleeping a challenge, so less of a woman's time in bed is actually spent sleeping. As a result, fatigue increases (see "Getting a good night's sleep during pregnancy," below). After giving birth, women are often exhausted. Not only are they at the mercy of their newborn's erratic sleep schedule, but breastfeeding also promotes sleepiness. Some research suggests that sleep disturbances during and after pregnancy may contribute to postpartum depression.

Getting a good night's sleep during pregnancy

In a National Sleep Foundation poll, nearly eight in 10 women reported disturbed sleep during pregnancy. Here are some tips to help you get a better night's sleep when you're expecting:

✔ Avoid spicy, fried, or acidic foods (such as tomato products), which contribute to heartburn.

✔ If you have heartburn, raise the head of your bed by placing blocks under the bedposts.

✔ Prevent nausea by eating frequent snacks during the day.

✔ If you feel drowsy, take a midday nap.

✔ Exercise regularly to reduce leg cramps and improve sleep.

✔ Cut down on fluids before bedtime to reduce nighttime trips to the bathroom.

✔ Use pillows or special pregnancy cushions to support your abdomen.

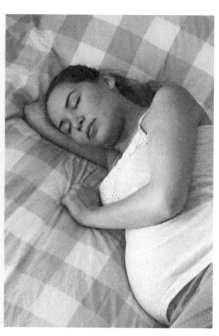

Thinkstock

Women who aren't pregnant may notice that their sleep habits shift throughout the month. During the second half of the menstrual cycle, progesterone levels rise, which tends to make women more drowsy than when levels are lower during the first half of the cycle. When both progesterone and estrogen levels fall a few days prior to menstruation, many women have trouble sleeping—one of the main symptoms of premenstrual syndrome, or PMS.

Middle age

As men and women enter middle age, deep sleep continues to diminish. Nighttime awakenings become more frequent and last longer. Waking after about three hours of sleep is particularly common. During menopause, many women experience hot flashes that can interrupt sleep. Obese people are more prone to nocturnal breathing problems, which often start during middle age. Men and women who are physically fit sleep more soundly as they grow older, compared with their sedentary peers.

The later years

In older adults, REM sleep decreases a small amount, but still hovers around 20% of total sleep time. Other changes are more pronounced. Deep sleep accounts for less than 10% of sleep time, and in some people it is completely absent. Falling asleep takes longer, and the shallow quality of sleep results in dozens of awakenings during the night. Doctors used to reassure older people that they needed less sleep than younger ones to function well, but sleep experts now know that isn't true. At any age, most adults need seven-and-a-half to eight hours of sleep to function at their best. Because of the frequent fragmentation of sleep, it can take longer in bed to get the same amount of sleep. If older people are unable to get all the required sleep at night, they often supplement nighttime sleep

A gene that affects circadian rhythms

Whether you're a night owl or an early riser, you probably know roughly how long you need to sleep to feel fully rested. Some people feel perky after just seven hours of sleep, while others are groggy if they log less than nine hours. The discovery of a genetic mutation in several people who need far less sleep than average helps explain at least some of this variation.

Scientists found the mutation in a gene called DEC2, which is known to affect circadian rhythms. The mutation occurred in a mother and daughter who were naturally short sleepers, requiring just six hours a night instead of the average of eight. Many Americans sleep just six hours nightly, but most rely on alarms, caffeine, and power naps to awaken and stay awake during the day. By contrast, these two women awoke naturally after six hours.

The scientists then created genetically engineered mice with the same mutation. The mice not only slept less and stayed awake longer, they also needed less sleep to recover following sleep deprivation.

The same researchers later discovered a different DEC2 mutation in fraternal twins, one with the mutation and one without. The twin with the mutation slept, on average, two hours less than his twin and needed far less time to recover from sleep deprivation. Now, an international team is sequencing other so-called CLOCK genes, which are involved in regulating circadian rhythms. The finding may help scientists better understand the nature of sleep and perhaps pave the way for new drugs to treat sleep disorders.

with daytime naps. This can be a successful strategy for accumulating sufficient total sleep over a 24-hour period. However, if you find that you need a nap, it's best to take one midday nap, rather than several brief ones scattered throughout the day and evening.

Sleep disturbances in elderly people, particularly in those who have Alzheimer's disease or other forms of dementia, are very disruptive for the individuals they affect and their caregivers. In one study, 70% of caregivers cited these problems as the decisive factor in seeking nursing home placement for a loved one. ♥

Dangers of sleep deprivation

Lack of sufficient sleep can lead to a range of ill effects, triggering mild to potentially life-threatening consequences, from weight gain to a heart attack (see Figure 4, below). Sleep deprivation is broadly categorized as complete or partial, based on duration and severity. Complete sleep deprivation happens when you pull an all-nighter. Partial sleep deprivation happens when you stint on sleep for a number of nights in a row (for example, only getting six hours of sleep each night for two weeks). But the mental and physical effects are similar.

Complete sleep deprivation

Normally, you're up for 16 or 17 hours before going to bed. As waking hours extend beyond this point, you first feel tired, then exhausted. Simple tasks that you would normally have no trouble accomplishing start to become difficult. In fact, a number of studies of hand-eye coordination and reaction time have shown that such sleep deprivation can be as debilitating as intoxication.

In one study, volunteers stayed awake for 28 hours (from 8 a.m. to noon the following day) and took tests of hand-eye coordination every 30 minutes during that time. On another day, the same volunteers completed the tests after drinking 10 to 15 grams of alcohol at 30-minute intervals until their blood alcohol content reached 0.10%—enough to be charged with driving while intoxicated in most states. The study concluded that 24 hours of wakefulness caused as much impairment as a blood alcohol content of 0.10%.

Sleep deprivation also leaves you prone to dozing off at the wheel and losing your concentration—two potentially dangerous phenomena that play a role in thousands of transportation accidents each year (see "Microsleeps and automatic behavior," page 11). When complete sleep deprivation extends for two or three days, people have difficulty completing tasks demanding a high attention level and often experience mood swings, depression, and increased feelings of tension. Sleep deprivation is so debilitating that it is sometimes used as a component of military interrogation.

Performance is also highly influenced by fluctuations in circadian rhythms. For example, sleep-deprived people may still function fairly well during the morning and evening. But during the peaks of sleepiness in the afternoon and overnight hours, people often literally cannot stay awake and may fall asleep while standing, sitting, or even while talking on the tele-

Figure 4: Health consequences of insufficient sleep

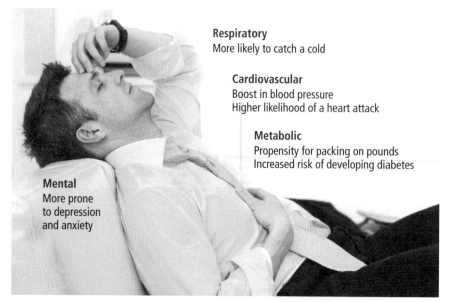

Respiratory
More likely to catch a cold

Cardiovascular
Boost in blood pressure
Higher likelihood of a heart attack

Metabolic
Propensity for packing on pounds
Increased risk of developing diabetes

Mental
More prone
to depression
and anxiety

People who skimp on sleep face a higher risk of numerous health problems.

phone, working on the computer, or eating. A small percentage experience paranoia and hallucinations.

Partial sleep deprivation

Partial sleep deprivation occurs when you get some sleep, but not 100% of what you need. Experts refer to this as building up a sleep debt.

After a single night of short sleep, most people function at or near their normal level. They may not feel great, but they can usually get through the day without others noticing that anything is amiss. After two or more nights of short sleep, people usually show signs of irritability and sleepiness. Work performance begins to suffer—particularly on complicated tasks—and people are more likely to complain of headaches, stomach problems, sore joints, memory lapses, and sluggish reaction time. In addition, people face a far higher risk of falling asleep on the job or while driving.

Long-term partial sleep deprivation occurs when someone gets less than the optimal amount of sleep

▶ **Microsleeps and automatic behavior**

Microsleeps are brief episodes of sleep that occur in the midst of ongoing wakeful activity. They can happen in people who are sleep deprived, often without their awareness. These are the head nods some people experience when trying to stay awake during a lecture, for example. They usually last just a few seconds but can go on for 10 or 15 seconds—and pose a grave danger if they happen when a person is driving. Brain-wave monitoring by EEG of someone experiencing microsleeps shows brief periods of stage N1 sleep intruding into wakefulness. During this time, the brain does not respond to noise or other sensory inputs, and you don't react to things happening around you. Because people are poor judges of when microsleeps will occur (and are equally poor at preventing them), they're a major factor in many motor vehicle accidents.

Automatic behavior refers to a period of several minutes or more during which a person is awake and performing routine duties but not attending to his or her surroundings or responding to changes in the environment. Examples include a driver who keeps the car on the road but misses an intended exit and a train engineer who can continue pressing a lever at regular intervals but doesn't notice an obstruction on the track.

for months or years on end—a common scenario for insomniacs and people with sleep disorders. But even healthy people who can't resist the round-the-clock commerce, communication, and entertainment opportunities our 24/7 society now offers may fall prey to this problem.

The health consequences may be serious. In a landmark study of human sleep deprivation, researchers followed a group of student volunteers who slept only four hours nightly for six consecutive days. The volunteers developed higher blood pressure and higher levels of the stress hormone cortisol, and they produced only half the usual number of antibodies to a flu vaccine. The sleep-deprived students also showed signs of insulin resistance—a condition that is the precursor of type 2 diabetes. All these changes—which were reversed when the students made up the hours of lost sleep—help explain why ongoing sleep debt raises the risk of a number of health problems.

How long-term sleep loss harms your health

A growing number of studies have linked long-term sleep deficits with significant health problems.

Diabetes. A report in *Diabetes Care* found a sharp increase in the risk of type 2 diabetes in people with persistent insomnia. People who had insomnia for a year or longer and who slept less than five hours per night had three times the risk of type 2 diabetes compared with those who had no sleep complaints and who slept six or more hours nightly. As with overweight and obesity (which are also closely linked to type 2 diabetes), the underlying cause is thought to involve a disruption of the body's normal hormonal regulation, but in this case, it results from insufficient sleep.

High blood pressure. Researchers involved in the diabetes study also evaluated risk of high blood pressure among the same group of people, which included more than 1,700 randomly chosen men and women from rural Pennsylvania. As described in the journal *Sleep*, the researchers found the risk of high blood pressure was three-and-a-half times greater among insomniacs who routinely slept less than six hours per night compared with normal sleepers who slept six or more hours nightly.

Heart disease. A number of studies have linked sleep deprivation with several well-known risk factors for heart disease, including higher cholesterol levels, higher triglyceride levels, and higher blood pressure. People who don't get sufficient sleep also have higher blood levels of stress hormones and substances that indicate inflammation, a key player in cardiovascular disease. Some research suggests that chronic sleep deprivation (getting no more than four hours a night) may double a woman's risk of dying of heart disease.

One common cause of poor sleep, sleep apnea (see "Obstructive sleep apnea," page 31) also raises heart disease risk. The low oxygen and high carbon dioxide levels that occur in apnea-disturbed sleep raise levels of stress hormones. This boosts blood pressure and heart rate, putting stress on the cardiovascular system. Sleep apnea appears to increase the risk of heart attack, heart failure, and heart rhythm disorders such as atrial fibrillation. People with moderate to severe sleep apnea have three times the risk of stroke compared with people who don't have the condition.

In the Wisconsin Sleep Cohort study, people with severe sleep apnea were three times more likely to die of heart disease during 18 years of follow-up than those without apnea. When researchers excluded those who used a breathing machine (a common apnea treatment), the risk jumped to more than five times higher. Apnea spells can trigger arrhythmias (irregular heartbeats), and the condition also increases the risk of stroke and heart failure.

Mental illness. A study of about 1,000 adults ages 21 to 30 found that, compared with normal sleepers, those who reported a history of insomnia during an interview were four times as likely to develop major depression by the time of a second interview three years later. And two studies in young people—one involving 300 pairs of young twins, and another including about 1,000 teenagers—found that sleep problems often developed before a diagnosis of major depression and (to a lesser extent) anxiety. Sleep problems in the teenagers preceded depression 69% of the time and anxiety disorders 27% of the time.

Viral infections. Anecdotal evidence supports the notion that when you're tired and run-down, you're more likely to get sick. A study in *Archives of Internal Medicine* offers some proof. Researchers tracked the sleep habits of 153 men and women for two weeks, then quarantined them for five days and exposed them to cold viruses. People who slept an average of less than seven hours per night were three times as likely to get sick as those who averaged at least eight hours.

Weight gain. Not getting enough sleep makes you more likely to gain weight, according to a review article in the journal *Obesity* that analyzed findings from 36 studies. The link appears to be especially strong among children. Lack of sufficient sleep tends to disrupt hormones that control hunger and appetite, and the resulting daytime fatigue often discourages you from exercising. Excess weight, in turn, increases the risk of a number of health problems—including some of those listed above. ◆

Practical tips for sounder sleep

Getting enough sleep is just as important as other vital elements of good health, such as eating a healthy diet, getting regular exercise, and practicing good dental hygiene. In short, sleep is not a luxury but a basic component of a healthy lifestyle. But just like purchasing healthy foods, taking an after-dinner walk, or flossing your teeth, getting adequate sleep requires time and discipline. Mentally block off certain hours for sleep and then follow through on your intention, avoid building up a sleep debt, and take steps to set up an ideal sleep environment. Seek a doctor's help if conventional steps toward good sleep don't work.

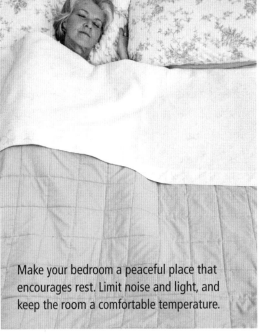

Make your bedroom a peaceful place that encourages rest. Limit noise and light, and keep the room a comfortable temperature.

Thinkstock

This doesn't mean that you can't have any fun, or that you need to get eight hours of sleep 365 days a year. Just as an occasional ice cream sundae won't make you fat, staying up a few extra hours for a party or to meet a deadline is perfectly acceptable—as long as you make plans to compensate the next day by taking a short afternoon nap or going to bed earlier. But over the long haul, you need to make sure you consistently get enough sleep.

Following are some ways to improve your sleep. These good habits are known as "sleep hygiene," because they represent scientific thinking about maintaining healthy sleep patterns.

Create a sleep sanctuary

A sleep-friendly bedroom can make it easier to fall and stay asleep, so take time to address issues that affect what you hear, see, and feel while in bed.

Control noise. A quiet bedroom is especially important for older adults, who spend less time in deep sleep. As a result, they are more easily awakened by noises. Here are some ways to reduce or disguise noises that can interfere with sleep:

- Decorate with heavy curtains and rugs, which absorb sounds.
- Install double-paned windows.
- Use earplugs.
- Use a fan or a sleep machine, which provide "white noise," or a recording of soothing sounds, such as falling rain, croaking frogs, or chirping crickets.

Dim bright light. Bright light at night can suppress your body's production of melatonin and make it harder to sleep. Keep your pre-bedtime light intake down with these steps:

- Avoid watching television or using a computer after 9 p.m.
- Don't read from a backlit electronic device (such as an iPad) at night.
- Replace bright lights with lower-wattage bulbs, or install dimmer switches that allow you to keep the lights low at night.

Bright bathroom lights can be an issue, especially since most people use the bathroom right before retiring (and sometimes in the middle of the night). But you don't want to stumble if you can't see. As long as it's safe to do so, consider using night-lights to light the way to and in your bathroom.

Keep comfortable. A bedroom that's too hot or too cold may interfere with sleep. Most people sleep best in a slightly cool room (around 65° F). Replace your mattress and pillows if they're worn or uncomfortable. If aching joints are keeping you awake, ask your doctor about pain relievers. Some people say they are more comfortable sleeping on "memory foam" mattresses and pillows (for example, Tempur-Pedic). See "Musculoskeletal disorders" on page 17 for advice on sleeping positions if you have specific joint pain.

Try relaxation rituals

Worrying about a problem or a long to-do list can be a recipe for insomnia. Well before you turn in, try writing down your worries and make a list of tasks you want to remember. This "worry journal" may help move these distracting thoughts from your mind.

Closer to bedtime, try comforting rituals that may help lull you to sleep:

- Listen to soft, calming music.
- Take a warm bath.
- Do some easy stretches.
- Read a book or magazine by soft light.

Once you crawl between the sheets, relaxation techniques (see page 22) can help you calm your body and mind. Mindfulness meditation has also proven helpful for battling insomnia. This type of meditation involves focusing on your breathing and then bringing your mind's attention to the present without drifting into concerns about the past or future. To learn more about mindfulness medita-

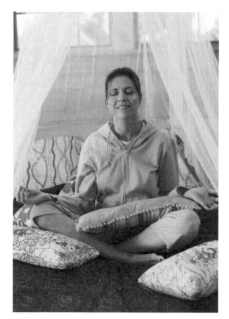

Relaxation techniques can help you calm your mind and body. Mindfulness meditation has proven helpful for insomnia.

tion, try one of the free guided recordings by Dr. Ronald Siegel, an assistant professor of psychology at Harvard Medical School and faculty editor of the Harvard Special Health Report *Positive Psychology*. The recordings are available at www.mindfulness-solution.com.

Stick to a schedule

A regular sleep schedule keeps the circadian sleep/wake cycle synchronized. People with the most regular sleep habits report the fewest problems with insomnia and the least depression. Experts advise getting up at about the same time every day, even after a late-night party or fitful sleep.

Limit the time you spend in bed. If you don't fall asleep within 20 minutes or if you wake up and can't fall back to sleep within that amount of time, get out of bed and do something relaxing until you feel sleepy again. Regardless of how well (or poorly) you slept, get out of bed at your regular time each morning to keep your circadian cycle synchronized.

Negotiate naps, if needed

If your goal is to sleep longer at night, napping is a bad idea. Your total daily sleep need stays constant, so naps take away from evening sleep. But if your goal is to be more alert during the day, a nap built into your daily schedule may be just the thing. If you have insomnia and feel anxious about getting enough sleep, then a sched-

Thinkstock

uled nap may help you sleep better at night by alleviating that anxiety.

If possible, nap shortly after lunch. People who snooze later in the afternoon tend to fall into a deeper sleep, which causes greater disruption at night. An ideal nap lasts no longer than an hour, and even a 15- to 20-minute nap has significant alertness benefits. Shorten or eliminate naps that produce lingering grogginess.

Keep a sleep diary

A sleep diary may help you uncover clues about what's disturbing your sleep. For example, you may realize that certain habits (like what you eat or drink or when you exercise) are affecting your slumber.

To keep a sleep diary, note what time you went to bed and woke up every day—preferably for two weeks to a month. Include entries for any medications you took, time and quantity of caffeine or alcohol consumption, when and how long you exercised, and any stresses you encountered during the day. All of these can affect sleep. Also note how well you slept each night, whether you awakened during the night, and, if so, for how long.

Curb caffeine

Caffeine, which is found in coffee, tea, sodas, and other beverages (see Table 2, at right), keeps you awake by blocking adenosine, a brain chemical that helps you fall asleep. For some people, a single cup of coffee in the morning means

a sleepless night. Caffeine can also interrupt sleep by increasing your need to get up to urinate at night.

If you have insomnia, avoid caffeine as much as possible, since its effects can last for many hours. Because caffeine withdrawal can cause headaches, irritability, and extreme fatigue, some people find it easier to cut back gradually than to go cold turkey. Those who can't or don't want to give up caffeine should avoid it after 2 p.m., or noon if they are especially caffeine-sensitive.

Nix nightcaps

Alcohol depresses the nervous system, so an alcoholic drink can help some people fall asleep. But the sleep won't necessarily be very good. Alcohol suppresses REM sleep, and the soporific effects disappear after a few hours. Drink-

ers have frequent awakenings and sometimes frightening dreams. Alcohol is responsible for up to 10% of chronic insomnia cases. Also, because alcohol relaxes throat muscles and interferes with brain control mechanisms, it can worsen snoring and other nocturnal breathing problems, sometimes to a dangerous extent.

Drinking during one of the body's intrinsic sleepy times—midafternoon or at night—will make a person more drowsy than imbibing at other times of day. Even one drink can make a sleep-deprived person drowsy. If you're driving a car, the combination significantly increases your chances of having an accident.

Quit tobacco

Nicotine is a potent stimulant that speeds your heart rate, raises

Table 2: Caffeine content in common drinks		
DRINK	SERVING SIZE	CAFFEINE (MILLIGRAMS)
Starbucks coffee	12 ounces	260
5-hour Energy	1.9 ounces	208
Monster Energy, Rockstar	16 ounces	160
Lipton Pure Leaf Iced Tea	18.5 ounces	60
Coca-Cola, Coke Zero, or Diet Pepsi	12 ounces	35
Decaf coffee from Dunkin' Donuts, Panera, or Starbucks	16 ounces	15 to 25
Lipton decaffeinated tea, brewed, black or green	8 ounces	5
7-Up or Sprite	12 ounces	0
Source: Center for Science in the Public Interest.		

blood pressure, and stimulates fast brain-wave activity that keeps you awake. If you're addicted to nicotine, a few hours without it is enough to induce withdrawal symptoms; the craving can even wake a smoker at night. People who kick the habit fall asleep more quickly and wake less often during the night. Sleep disturbance and daytime fatigue may occur during the initial withdrawal from nicotine. But even during this period, many former users report improvements in sleep. If you continue to use tobacco, avoid smoking or chewing it for at least one to two hours before bedtime.

Energize with exercise (but not at night)

Walking, jogging, swimming, or any type of exercise that gets your heart pumping faster provides three important sleep benefits: you fall asleep faster, you spend more time in deep sleep, and you awaken less often during the night. Exercise seems to be of particular benefit to older people. In one study, physically fit older men fell asleep in less than half the time it took for sedentary men, and they woke up less often during the night.

Studies also suggest that even gentle exercise, such as stretching and toning, can help people sleep better. Consider trying yoga or tai chi, a stylized martial arts practice that features a series of slow, flowing motions and deep, slow breathing.

Exercise is the only known way for healthy adults to boost the amount of deep sleep they get. Research shows that older men and women who report sleeping normally can still increase the amount of time they spend in deep sleep if they do some form of aerobic activity.

Exercising outdoors in the morning is ideal, because bright, natural daylight can help set your natural circadian rhythms. Try to avoid exercise within two hours of bedtime because exercise is stimulating and can make it harder to fall asleep.

Watch when and what you eat and drink

A grumbling stomach can be distracting enough to keep you awake, so if you're hungry right before bed, eat a small healthy snack, such as an apple with a slice of cheese or a few whole-wheat crackers, to satisfy you until breakfast.

But an overly full belly may be even more disrupting. Avoid eating a big meal within two to three hours of bedtime. And steer clear of foods that contribute to acid reflux (heartburn), as lying down can provoke or worsen the problem. Common culprits include coffee, chocolate, alcohol, peppermint, and fatty foods. If you're prone to acid reflux, elevate your upper body with an under-mattress wedge or blocks placed under the bedposts. Over-the-counter and prescription drugs that suppress stomach acid secretion can also help. Finally, if you sleep on your right side, try to sleep on your left side instead, as several studies suggest that sleeping on your right side aggravates heartburn.

Even if you're careful to avoid caffeinated or alcoholic beverages, drinking too much of any fluid too close to bedtime may cause you to wake up to use the bathroom. ◗

Medical conditions that disrupt sleep

People who feel they sleep perfectly well may still be troubled by excessive daytime sleepiness because of a variety of underlying medical illnesses. Common conditions often associated with sleep problems include diabetes, heart disease, musculoskeletal disorders, kidney disease, mental illness, neurological disorders, respiratory problems, and thyroid disease. The stress of chronic illness can also cause insomnia and daytime drowsiness. In addition, a number of prescription and over-the-counter medications used to treat these and other health problems can impair sleep quality and quantity (see Table 3, page 18).

Diabetes

Night sweats, a frequent need to urinate, or symptoms of hypoglycemia (low blood sugar) often rouse people with diabetes whose blood sugar levels are not well controlled. Tight glucose control will reduce these symptoms. If diabetes has damaged nerves in the legs, nighttime movements or pain may also disturb sleep and require medication for relief and to improve sleep.

Heart disease

People with heart failure may awaken during the night feeling short of breath because extra body fluid accumulates around their lungs when they're lying down. Placing blocks under the head of the bed to elevate the upper body may help. These people can also be awakened just as they are falling asleep by a characteristic breathing pattern called Cheyne-Stokes respiration, a series of increasingly deep breaths followed by a brief cessation of breathing. Benzodiazepine sleep medications (see "Prescription medications for insomnia," page 23) help some people stay asleep, but others may need to use supplemental oxygen or a device that increases pressure in the upper airway and chest cavity (see "Treatments for obstructive sleep apnea," page 32).

People with heart failure frequently also have obstructive sleep apnea, which can disrupt sleep, cause

snooze news | The National Center on Sleep Disorders Research estimates that each year, sleep disorders, sleep deprivation, and sleepiness add $15.9 billion to the national health care bill. And that doesn't include costs to society for related health problems, such as lost worker productivity and accidents. A report in the journal *Sleep* estimated that lost work productivity due to insomnia costs the United States $63.2 billion per year. Insomnia-related work accidents cost about $31 billion per year, according to a study in *Archives of General Psychiatry*.

daytime sleepiness, and worsen heart failure. In people with coronary artery disease, the natural fluctuations in hormone secretion reflecting circadian rhythms may trigger angina (chest pain), arrhythmia (irregular heartbeat), or even a heart attack while asleep.

Musculoskeletal disorders

Arthritis pain can make it hard for people to fall asleep and to resettle when they shift positions. In addition, treatment with corticosteroids frequently causes insomnia. You may find it helpful to take aspirin or a nonsteroidal anti-inflammatory drug (NSAID) just before bedtime, but because of potential side effects, check with your doctor before taking it regularly. For specific joint issues, try these sleeping positions:

- **Neck:** Sleep with a single flat pillow to place the neck in the most neutral position, avoiding extremes of rotation and sideways bending. Avoid sleeping on your stomach; instead, sleep on your back or side.
- **Low back:** Sleep on your back or side with your knees and hips both flexed to about 90 degrees. This position can relieve pressure on lumbar discs for people with degenerative disc disease or disc herniation. Use a heating pad at bedtime to relieve pain.
- **Knee:** Sleep with a pillow between your legs to reduce strain on the joint.
- **Hip:** Sleep on your side with a pillow between your

Table 3: Medications that may affect sleep

A number of drugs steal sleep, while others may cause unwanted drowsiness. Your doctor may be able to suggest alternatives that do not disrupt sleep.

MEDICATION	USED TO TREAT	COMMON EXAMPLES	POSSIBLE EFFECT ON SLEEP AND DAYTIME FUNCTIONING
Beta blockers*	High blood pressure, heart rhythm problems, angina	metoprolol (Lopressor), pindolol (Visken), propranolol (Inderal)	Insomnia, nighttime awakenings, nightmares
Clonidine	High blood pressure; sometimes prescribed off-label for alcohol withdrawal, smoking cessation, or other health problems	clonidine (Catapres)	Daytime drowsiness and fatigue, disrupted REM sleep; less commonly, restlessness, early morning awakening, nightmares
Corticosteroids	Inflammation, asthma	prednisone (Sterapred, others)	Daytime jitters, insomnia, decreased REM sleep
Diuretics	High blood pressure	chlorothiazide (Diuril), chlorthalidone (Hygroton), hydrochlorothiazide (Esidrix, HydroDiuril, others)	Increased nighttime urination, painful calf cramps during sleep
Medications containing alcohol	Cough, cold, and flu	Contact Cold and Flu, Nyquil Cough, many others	Suppressed REM sleep, disrupted nighttime sleep
Medications containing caffeine	Decreased alertness	Caffedrine, NoDoz, Vivarin	Wakefulness that may last up to six to seven hours
	Headaches and other pain	Anacin, Excedrin, Midol	
Nicotine replacement products	Smoking	nicotine patches (Nicoderm), gum (Nicorette), nasal spray or inhalers (Nicotrol), and lozenges (Commit)	Insomnia, disturbing dreams
Sedating antihistamines**	Cold and allergy symptoms	chlorpheniramine (Chlor-Trimeton), diphenhydramine (Benadryl)	Drowsiness
	Motion sickness	dimenhydrinate (Dramamine)	
Selective serotonin reuptake inhibitors (SSRIs)	Depression, anxiety	fluoxetine (Prozac), paroxetine (Paxil), sertraline (Zoloft)	Decreased REM sleep, daytime fatigue
Sympathomimetic stimulants	Attention deficit disorder	dextroamphetamine and amphetamine (Adderall), methylphenidate (Ritalin, Concerta)	Difficulty falling asleep, decreased REM and non-REM deep sleep
Theophylline	Asthma, chronic obstructive pulmonary disease (COPD)	theophylline (Slo-bid, Theo-Dur, others)	Wakefulness similar to that caused by caffeine
Thyroid hormone	Hypothyroidism	levothyroxine (Levoxyl, Synthroid, others)	Difficulty falling asleep, fragmented sleep, insomnia (at higher doses)

*Some beta blockers do not affect sleep; they include atenolol (Tenormin) and sotalol (Betapace).

**These medications are also found in over-the-counter sleep aids.

legs, or sleep on your back to avoid a position that rotates the hip.

People with fibromyalgia—a condition characterized by painful ligaments and tendons—are likely to wake in the morning still feeling fatigued and as stiff and achy as a person with arthritis. Researchers who analyzed the sleep of fibromyalgia sufferers have found that at least half have abnormal deep sleep, in which slow (delta) brain waves are mixed with faster (alpha) waves that are usually associated with relaxed wakefulness, a pattern called alpha-delta sleep. In one study, 62 people with fibromyalgia received treatment for six weeks with either the NSAID naproxen, the tricyclic antidepressant amitriptyline, both drugs, or a placebo. Almost half of those who took low doses of amitriptyline reported sleeping and feeling better.

Kidney disease

Kidney disease can cause waste products to build up in the blood and can result in insomnia or symptoms of restless legs syndrome. Although researchers aren't sure why, kidney dialysis or transplant does not always return sleep to normal.

Mental illness

Almost all people with anxiety or depression have trouble falling asleep and staying asleep. In turn, not being able to sleep may become a focus of ongoing fear and tension, causing further sleep loss.

General anxiety. Severe anxiety, formally known as generalized anxiety disorder, is a mental illness characterized by persistent, nagging feelings of worry, apprehension, or uneasiness. These feelings are either unusually intense or out of proportion to the real troubles and dangers of the person's everyday life. People with the disorder typically experience excessive, persistent worry every day or almost every day for a period of six months or more. Common symptoms include trouble falling asleep, trouble staying asleep, and not feeling rested after sleep.

Phobias and panic attacks. Phobias, which are intense fears related to a specific object or situation, rarely cause sleep problems unless the phobia is itself sleep-related (such as fear of nightmares or of the bedroom). Panic attacks, on the other hand, often strike at night. In fact, the timing of nocturnal attacks helped convince psychiatrists that these episodes are biologically based. Sleep-related panic attacks do not occur during dreaming, but rather in stage N2 and deep sleep, which are free of psychological triggers. In many phobias and panic disorders, recognizing and treating the underlying problem—often with an anti-anxiety medication—may solve the sleep disturbance.

Depression. Because almost 90% of people with serious depression experience insomnia, a physician evaluating a person with insomnia will consider depression as a possible cause. Waking up too early in the morning is a hallmark of depression, and some depressed people have difficulty falling asleep or sleep fitfully throughout the whole night. In chronic, low-grade depression, insomnia or sleepiness may be the most prominent symptom. Laboratory studies have shown that people who are depressed spend less time in deep sleep and may enter REM sleep more quickly at the beginning of the night.

Bipolar disorder. Disturbed sleep is a prominent feature of bipolar disorder (manic-depressive illness). Sleep loss may worsen or induce manic symptoms or temporarily alleviate depression. During a manic episode, a person may not sleep at all for several days. Such occurrences are often followed by a "crash" during which the person spends most of the next few days in bed.

Coping with frequent nighttime urination

Nocturia—the need to get up frequently to urinate during the night—is a common cause of sleep loss, especially among older adults. It affects nearly two-thirds of adults ages 55 to 84 at least a few nights per week.

A mild case causes a person to wake up at least twice during the night; in severe cases, a person may get up as many as five or six times. Not surprisingly, this can lead to significant sleep deprivation and daytime fatigue.

Nocturia becomes more common with age. As you get older, your body produces less of an antidiuretic hormone called arginine vasopressin that enables you to retain fluid. With lower concentrations of this hormone, you produce more urine at night. Also, the bladder tends to lose holding capacity as you age, and older people are more likely to suffer from medical problems that affect the bladder.

Nocturia has numerous possible other causes, including some of the disorders mentioned in this report (heart failure, diabetes), other medical conditions (urinary tract infection, an enlarged prostate, liver failure, multiple sclerosis, sleep apnea), and medication (especially diuretics). Some cases are caused or worsened by excessive fluid intake after dinner, especially drinks containing alcohol or caffeine.

Therapies fall into three categories: behavioral interventions, medication, and treatments to correct medical causes. The first step is to try to identify the cause and correct it. If that doesn't work, behavioral approaches such as cutting down on how much you drink in the two hours before bedtime, especially caffeine and alcohol, may do the trick. If the nocturia persists, your doctor may prescribe a drug to treat an overactive bladder. The most commonly used is desmopressin (DDAVP, Stimate), which mimics some of the action of the antidiuretic hormone. If the problem stems from increased contractions of the bladder, relaxant agents such as tolterodine (Detrol) and oxybutynin (Ditropan, Oxytrol) can help.

Schizophrenia. Some people with schizophrenia sleep very little when they enter an acute phase of their illness. Between episodes, their sleep patterns are likely to improve, although many schizophrenics rarely obtain a normal amount of deep sleep.

Other neurological disorders

Certain brain and nerve disorders can contribute to sleeplessness.

Dementia. Alzheimer's disease and other forms of dementia may disrupt sleep regulation and other brain functions. Wandering, disorientation, and agitation during the evening and night, a phenomenon known as "sundowning," can require constant supervision and place great stress on caregivers. In such cases, small doses of antipsychotic medications such as haloperidol (Haldol) and thioridazine (Mellaril) are more helpful than benzodiazepine drugs.

Epilepsy. People with epilepsy are twice as likely as others to suffer from insomnia. Brain-wave disturbances that cause seizures can also cause deficits in deep sleep or REM sleep. Antiseizure drugs can cause similar changes at first, but tend to correct these sleep disturbances when used for a long time. About one in four people with epilepsy has seizures that occur mainly at night, causing disturbed sleep and daytime sleepiness. Sleep deprivation can also trigger a seizure, a phenomenon noted in college infirmaries during exam periods, as some students suffer their first seizures after staying up late to study.

Headaches, strokes, and tumors. People who are prone to headaches should try to avoid sleep deprivation, as lack of sleep can promote headaches. Both cluster headaches and migraines may be related to changes in the size of blood vessels leading to the cortex of the brain; pain occurs when the walls of the blood vessels dilate. Researchers theorize that as the body catches up on missed sleep, it spends more time in delta sleep, when vessels are most constricted, making the transition to REM sleep more dramatic and likely to induce a headache. Headaches that awaken people are often migraines, but some migraines can be relieved by sleep.

Sleepiness coupled with dizziness, weakness, headache, or vision problems may signal a serious problem such as a brain tumor or stroke, which requires immediate medical attention.

Parkinson's disease. Almost all people with Parkinson's disease have insomnia. Just getting in and out of bed can be a struggle, and the disease often disrupts sleep. Some arousals are from the tremors and movements caused by the disorder, and others seem to result from the disorder itself. Treatment with sleeping pills may be difficult because some drugs can worsen Parkinson's symptoms. Some people who take drugs such as levodopa, the mainstay of Parkinson's treatment, develop severe nightmares; others experience disruption of REM sleep. However, the use of these medications at night is important to maintain the mobility needed to change positions in bed. A bed rail or an overhead bar (known as a trapeze) may make it easier for people with Parkinson's to move about and, therefore, lead to better sleep.

Respiratory problems

Circadian-related changes in the tone of the muscles surrounding the airways can cause the airways to constrict during the night, raising the potential for nocturnal asthma attacks that rouse the sleeper abruptly. Breathing difficulties or fear of having an attack may make it more difficult to fall asleep, as can the use of steroids, theophylline, or other breathing medications that also have a stimulating effect, similar to that of caffeine. One study found that nearly 75% of people with asthma experienced frequent awakenings every week. People who have emphysema or bronchitis may also have difficulty falling and staying asleep because of excess sputum production, shortness of breath, and coughing.

Thyroid disease

An overactive thyroid (hyperthyroidism) overstimulates the nervous system, making it hard to fall asleep, and may cause night sweats, leading to nighttime arousals. Feeling cold and sleepy is a hallmark of an underactive thyroid (hypothyroidism). Because thyroid function affects every organ and system in the body, the symptoms can be wide-ranging and sometimes difficult to decipher. Checking thyroid function requires only a simple blood test, so if you notice a variety of unexplained symptoms, ask your doctor for a thyroid test. ◆

Insomnia

If you suffer from insomnia, you may be plagued by trouble falling asleep, unwelcome awakenings during the night, and fitful sleep. You may feel drowsy during the day, yet still be unable to nap. You may frequently be anxious, irritable, forgetful, and unable to concentrate.

Although it's the most common sleep disturbance, insomnia is not a single disorder, but rather a general symptom like fever or pain. Finding a remedy requires uncovering the cause. Nearly half of insomnia cases stem from psychological or emotional problems. Stressful events, mild depression, or an anxiety disorder can keep you awake at night. With proper treatment of the underlying cause, the insomnia usually recedes. If it doesn't, additional treatment focusing on sleep may help. The two main approaches to treating insomnia—behavioral therapy and medications—are both effective. But behavioral therapy has proven to be longer lasting and doesn't have the side effects that can occur with medications.

Types of insomnia

One way doctors classify insomnia is by its duration. Insomnia is considered transient if it lasts only a few days, short-term if it continues for a few weeks, and chronic if the problem persists.

The causes of transient or short-term insomnia are usually apparent to the sufferer—the death of or separation from a loved one, nervousness about an upcoming event (such as a wedding, public speaking engagement, or move), jet lag, or discomfort from an illness or injury. Chronic insomnia may be caused by a number of medications or medical conditions (see "Medical conditions that disrupt sleep," page 17). In these instances, treating the condition or changing the medication may relieve the insomnia.

One common form of persistent sleeplessness is conditioned (learned) insomnia. After experiencing a few sleepless nights, some people learn to associate the bedroom with being awake. Taking steps to compensate for sleep deprivation—napping, drinking coffee, having a nightcap, or forgoing exercise—only fuels the problem. As insomnia worsens, anxiety regarding the insomnia may also worsen, leading to a vicious cycle in which fears about sleeplessness and its consequences become the primary cause of the insomnia.

First-line treatment: Behavioral changes

For chronic insomnia, the treatment of choice is behavioral therapy, which uses a variety of behavioral techniques, such as changing your lifestyle and habits, to improve sleep. A careful evaluation can pinpoint habits that keep you up at night. A sleep specialist trained in behavioral medicine can help people with learned insomnia replace their bad habits with positive ones.

Sleep restriction

People with insomnia often spend more time in bed, hoping this will lead to sleep. In reality, spending *less* time in bed—a technique known as sleep restriction—promotes more restful sleep and helps make the bedroom a welcome sight instead of a torture chamber. As you learn to fall asleep quickly and sleep soundly, the time in bed is slowly extended until you obtain a full night's sleep.

Some sleep experts suggest starting with six hours at first, or whatever amount of time you typically sleep at night. Setting a rigid early morning waking time often works best. If the alarm is set for 7 a.m., a six-hour restriction means that no matter how sleepy you are, you must stay awake until 1 a.m. Once you are sleeping well during the allotted six hours, you can add another 15 or 30 minutes, then repeat the process until you're getting a healthy amount of sleep.

Stimulus control

Developed in the 1970s, this technique (also known as reconditioning) trains people with insomnia to associate the bedroom with sleep instead of sleeplessness and frustration. These are the rules:

- Use the bed only for sleeping or sex.
- Don't spend time in bed not sleeping. Go to bed only when you're sleepy. If you're unable to sleep, move to another room and do something relaxing. Stay up until you are sleepy, then return to bed. If sleep does not follow quickly, repeat.
- During the reconditioning process, get up at the same time every day and do not nap, regardless of how much sleep you got the night before.

Relaxation techniques

For some people with insomnia, a racing or worried mind is the enemy of sleep. In others, physical tension is to blame. Techniques to quiet a racing mind—such as meditation, breathing exercises, progressive muscle relaxation, and biofeedback—can be learned in behavior therapy sessions or from books or classes.

Progressive muscle relaxation, which involves progressively tensing and relaxing your muscles starting with your feet and working your way up your body, is a tried-and-true, drug-free technique for achieving both physical and mental relaxation. A typical approach is this:

- Lie on your back in a comfortable position. Put a pillow under your head if you like, or place one under your knees to relax your back. Rest your arms, with palms up, slightly apart from your body. Feel your shoulders relax.
- Take several slow, deep breaths through your nose. Exhale with a long sigh to release tension.
- Focus on your feet and ankles. Are they painful or tense? Tighten the muscles briefly to feel the sensation. Let your feet sink into the floor or the bed. Feel them getting heavy and becoming totally relaxed. Let them drop from your consciousness.
- Slowly move your attention through different parts of your body: your calves, thighs, lower back, hips, and pelvic area; your middle back, abdomen, upper back, shoulders, arms, and hands; your neck, jaw, tongue, forehead, and scalp. Feel your body relax

▶ Gadgets that promise better sleep: Worth a try?

In recent years, a number of smartphone apps, gadgets, and specialized devices that pledge to deliver a more satisfying slumber have hit the market, aimed directly to sleep-deprived consumers. They include a range of products, from wristband or mattress sensors that record your movement in bed to specialized lights that claim to either help you fall asleep or wake up.

Be aware that there's little research demonstrating the effectiveness of any of these products, which don't require a great deal of evidence to gain marketing approval. There are no known downsides to trying any of them, save for the cost (if any). If you try one but still have troubling symptoms, consult your health care provider.

and your lungs gently expand and contract. Relax any spots that are still tense. Breathe softly.

- If thoughts distract you, gently ignore them and return your attention to your breathing. Your worries and thoughts will be there when you are ready to acknowledge them.

Another way to release physical tension and relax more effectively is to use biofeedback. This approach involves using equipment that monitors involuntary body states (such as muscle tension or hand temperature) and makes you aware of them. Immediate feedback helps you see how various thoughts or relaxation maneuvers affect tension, enabling you to learn how to gain voluntary control over the process. Biofeedback is usually done under professional supervision.

Cognitive behavioral therapy

Cognitive behavioral therapy (CBT) teaches people new ways of thinking about and then doing things. CBT has proved helpful in treating addictions, phobias, and anxiety—as well as insomnia.

CBT for insomnia aims to change negative thoughts and beliefs about sleep into positive ones. People with insomnia tend to become preoccupied with sleep and apprehensive about the consequences of poor sleep. This worry makes relaxing and falling asleep nearly impossible—a phenomenon some experts refer to as "insomniaphobia." The basic tenets of this therapy include setting realistic goals and learning to let go of inaccurate thoughts that can interfere with sleep.

Here are some common types and examples of these thoughts:

- Misattributions: "When I feel nervous during the day, it's always because I did not sleep well the night before."
- Hopelessness: "I'll never get a decent night's rest."
- Unrealistic expectations: "I need eight hours of sleep tonight" or "I have to fall asleep before my spouse does."
- Exaggerating consequences: "If I don't get to sleep soon, I'll embarrass myself at tomorrow's meeting."
- Performance anxiety: "It will take me at least an hour to fall asleep."

A cognitive behavioral therapist helps you replace these maladaptive thoughts with accurate and constructive ones, such as "All my problems do not stem from insomnia," "I stand a good chance of getting a good night's sleep tonight," or "My job does not depend on how much sleep I get tonight." The therapist also provides structure and support while you practice new thoughts and habits. Typically, you meet with the therapist once a week for an hour, for six to eight weeks.

In recent years, CBT for insomnia has been refined, expanded, and dubbed "CBT-i." It includes teaching people the behavioral treatments explained above (sleep restriction, stimulus control, and relaxation) as well as the sleep hygiene techniques described earlier in this report (see "Practical tips for sounder sleep," page 13).

In a 2014 review article in *Annals of Internal Medicine*, researchers combined data from 20 different trials of CBT-i involving more than 1,100 people with chronic insomnia. On average, people treated with CBT-i fell asleep almost 20 minutes faster and spent 30 fewer minutes awake during the night compared with people who didn't undergo CBT-i.

These improvements are as good as, or better than, those seen in people who take prescription sleep medications such as zolpidem (Ambien) and eszopiclone (Lunesta). And unlike medications, the effects of CBT-i last even after the therapy ends—at least six months, according to one study. Medications, in contrast, stop working when you stop taking them.

The biggest obstacle to successful treatment with CBT-i is the commitment it requires. Some people fail to complete all the required sessions or to practice the techniques on their own. Internet-based programs might help address that problem. Several small studies suggest that online CBT-i programs that teach people good sleep hygiene, relaxation techniques, and other strategies can help insomniacs sleep better.

One such program, called SHUTi (Sleep Healthy Using the Internet), helped long-term insomniacs boost their sleep efficiency by an average of 16%, and participants were about half as likely to wake up after falling asleep, compared with a control group. Another study documented at least mild improvements in about 80% of people who completed five weeks of online CBT, with 35% reporting that their sleep was "much improved" or "very much improved." And a Scottish study, which used an automated virtual therapist, also showed clear improvements in sleep and daytime functioning in people with insomnia. The benefits largely persisted two months after the intervention.

Many health insurance plans cover CBT-i, which falls under mental health coverage. There's only one problem: not many therapists are trained in this specific type of talk therapy. Even in the medical mecca of Boston, only about five clinicians offer CBT-i. You can find lists of certified specialists throughout the country from the American Board of Sleep Medicine and the Society for Behavioral Sleep Medicine (see "Resources," page 52).

Prescription medications for insomnia

Prescription medications help some people with insomnia, but it's best to use them at the lowest effective dose and for the shortest possible period of time. These drugs are most appropriate for short-term problems that disrupt sleep, such as traveling across time zones or coping with a death in the family. For longer-term insomnia, behavioral therapies should be tried first, as they are often just as effective and may have longer-lasting benefits—without negative side effects.

Medications to treat insomnia (see Table 4, page 24) include benzodiazepines, which are also used to

Table 4: Prescription medications for insomnia

GENERIC NAME (BRAND NAME)	SIDE EFFECTS	COMMENTS
Benzodiazepines (for short-term treatment of insomnia)		
alprazolam* (Xanax) clonazepam* (Klonopin) diazepam* (Valium) estazolam (ProSom) flurazepam (Dalmane) lorazepam* (Ativan) quazepam (Doral) temazepam (Restoril) triazolam (Halcion)	Clumsiness or unsteadiness, dizziness, lightheadedness, daytime drowsiness, headache	Should be used with caution by people with sleep apnea or other breathing difficulties; not to be used with alcohol or other depressants; tolerance may develop; withdrawal symptoms occur if stopped abruptly. Triazolam is a short-acting medication.
Nonbenzodiazepines (for insomnia)		
eszopiclone (Lunesta) zaleplon (Sonata) zolpidem** (Ambien, Ambien CR)	Headache, daytime drowsiness, dizziness, nausea, drugged feeling	Don't take these medications with alcohol and certain depressants (including antihistamines, muscle relaxants, and sedatives).
Antidepressants (for insomnia, nonrestorative sleep, and depression)		
Serotonin modulator trazodone* (Desyrel)	Dizziness, dry mouth, headache, nausea, constipation or diarrhea, painful erections	Do not take with a monoamine oxidase inhibitor (MAOI) or while recovering from a heart attack.
Selective serotonin reuptake inhibitors (SSRIs) citalopram* (Celexa) fluoxetine* (Prozac) fluvoxamine* (Luvox) paroxetine* (Paxil) sertraline* (Zoloft)	Dry mouth, drowsiness, dizziness, sexual dysfunction, nausea, diarrhea, headache, jitteriness, sweating, insomnia, weight gain	
Serotonin and norepinephrine reuptake inhibitor (SNRI) venlafaxine* (Effexor)	Upset stomach, excitement or anxiety, dry mouth, skin sensitivity to sunlight, weight gain, headache	
Tetracyclic mirtazapine* (Remeron)	Dry mouth, constipation, weight gain, headache, dizziness	
Tricyclics amitriptyline* (Elavil) doxepin (Sinequan,* Silenor) nortriptyline* (Aventyl, Pamelor) trimipramine* (Surmontil)	Dry mouth, dizziness, constipation, incomplete urination, weight gain, sun sensitivity, sweating, faintness upon standing, increased heart rate, sexual dysfunction	
Melatonin-receptor agonist (for insomnia at bedtime)		
ramelteon (Rozerem)	Dizziness	May exacerbate depression; not to be used by people who have severe liver damage or who take fluvoxamine (Luvox).
Orexin-receptor antagonist		
suvorexant (Belsomra)	Dizziness, headache, unusual dreams, dry mouth, cough	New medication, so full range of side effects not yet known.

Although the FDA has not approved these drugs for insomnia, physicians have found that they often help people with insomnia and therefore prescribe them. The only antidepressant with FDA approval for insomnia is Silenor. (Sinequan has the same active ingredient, but it does not have approval for this use.)

**See "Nonbenzodiazepines," page 25, for a description of the different formulations of this medication.*

treat anxiety; related medications known as nonbenzodiazepines, which selectively target sleep receptors in the brain; and antidepressants, which are typically prescribed in doses lower than those used to treat depression. Two newer sleep drugs target two different brain chemicals—melatonin and orexin—involved in sleep regulation.

Benzodiazepines

These medications enhance the activity of GABA, a neurotransmitter that calms brain activity. Different benzodiazepines vary in how quickly they take effect and how long they remain active in the body. Taken at night, benzodiazepines can lead to next-day drowsiness and sedation. If your main problem is getting to sleep, your doctor may prescribe one that begins working quickly and is short-acting, such as triazolam (Halcion). If your problem is staying asleep, a drug that lasts longer—such as estazolam (ProSom) or temazepam (Restoril)—may be necessary. These drugs are useful for people with anxiety and insomnia that results from it.

One drawback of benzodiazepines is that they reduce how much deep sleep you get. Also, many people who use benzodiazepines develop tolerance—the need for more and more of the drug to obtain the same effect. After a few weeks, the drugs may no longer promote sleep. Another risk is that stopping the medication abruptly after using it for months can cause insomnia that's even worse than the insomnia you had before you started taking the drug (a phenomenon known as rebound). These medications should be discontinued under a doctor's supervision because withdrawal may lead to muscle tension, restlessness, irritability, or, in rare cases, convulsions.

Nonbenzodiazepines

These medications also enhance the sleep-inducing activity of GABA, but they have a slightly different chemical composition. While benzodiazepines affect a range of different receptors in the brain, the nonbenzodiazepines act only on the sleep receptors, which means they cause fewer side effects. They also appear to have little or no effect on deep sleep. Many physicians now prescribe these drugs—which include eszopiclone (Lunesta), zaleplon (Sonata), and zolpidem (Ambien)—in situations where they used to prescribe benzodiazepines.

All three drugs make you fall asleep quicker, but only eszopiclone and zolpidem lengthen total sleep time. Zaleplon and zolpidem act quickly (within 20 minutes) and, for the most part, wear off before your typical waking time. Zaleplon wears off especially quickly, so it may not keep you asleep the whole night if you take it before bed. But you can take one if you wake up in the middle of the night and can't fall back asleep. Eszopiclone takes a little longer to take effect and also lasts longer. A long-acting version of zolpidem, called Ambien CR, helps with problems with staying asleep as well as falling asleep.

Zolpidem also comes as a tablet you place under your tongue (Edluar, Intermezzo) and an oral spray (Zolpimist), which you spray over your tongue. These new formulations are absorbed more quickly, so they may take effect sooner—and are easier to use because you don't need water to take them. Intermezzo contains a lower dose of zolpidem (less than half of the amount in an Ambien tablet), so it wears off in about four hours—a benefit for those who wake up in the middle of the night and need help to fall back asleep. In fact, Intermezzo is the only prescription sleep medication approved for middle-of-the-night awakening.

However, there are drawbacks to zolpidem. Researchers at the Mayo Clinic in Rochester, Minn., found that hospitalized people who take Ambien have four times the risk of falls compared with those who don't take the sleep aid. The findings, published in the *Journal of Hospital Medicine*, prompted the Mayo Clinic to phase out its use of Ambien (which is commonly used in hospitals) and rely more on nondrug methods to promote sleep. These include emphasizing quiet, reducing interruptions, and helping people use techniques such as progressive muscle relaxation, guided imagery, and breathing exercises. Guidance on some of these techniques is available via video in hospital rooms.

In early 2013, the FDA warned that people who take zolpidem can wake up the next morning with drug levels high enough to impair their ability to drive and do other activities safely—even if they feel wide awake. Experts originally believed zolpidem worked quickly and left the body quickly, too—but new data suggest it takes longer than previously thought for the drug to be eliminated. The highest risk is with the extended-release form (available as a generic or as Ambien CR). Women are particularly vulnerable because they clear zolpidem from their bodies more slowly than men do. All the other forms of zolpidem (except for Intermezzo) may cause the same problem. As a result, the agency has told manufacturers of these medications to lower the starting dose of products containing zolpidem, as follows:

Women: the 10-mg recommended dose for Ambien, Edluar, and Zolpimist should be cut in half to 5 mg; 12.5-mg doses of extended-release zolpidem (Ambien CR) should be cut in half to 6.25 mg.

Men: Clinicians should consider prescribing a 5-mg dose for regular zolpidem and a 6.25-mg dose for the extended-release form.

With any sleeping pill you take, allow for eight hours of sleep, and avoid doing things that demand high levels of alertness first thing in the morning.

While zolpidem and zaleplon are both approved only to treat short-term insomnia (for up to 30 days), eszopiclone is approved to treat insomnia for up to six months. This does not mean eszopiclone is necessarily superior—just that its manufacturer took the time and expense to conduct studies to show the drug is safe and effective for longer use.

While nonbenzodiazepines have fewer drawbacks than benzodiazepines, they're not perfect for everyone. Some people find the drugs aren't powerful enough to put them to sleep. And the drugs may still cause morning grogginess, tolerance, and rebound insomnia, as well as headache, dizziness, nausea, and, in rare cases, sleepwalking and sleep eating (see "Sleeping pills and sleep eating," above right). The long-term effects of nonbenzodiazepines remain unknown.

Antidepressants

Most of these medications are not approved for insomnia, except for doxepin (Silenor), which was originally developed as an antidepressant under the name Sinequan. Some doctors believe antidepressants have fewer side effects and are safer for long-term use

Sleeping pills and sleep eating

Several news reports in 2006 drew attention to a strange side effect of zolpidem (Ambien): sleep eating. People were seen foraging for food at night but were unable to remember the episodes in the morning, or they reported finding evidence of a midnight feast with no recollection of the event. Several people even gained quite a lot of weight.

Other unusual side effects seen with Ambien and related drugs include sleepwalking, short-term amnesia, and, rarely, sleep driving. Some of the driving cases occurred when people took sleep medication after drinking alcohol. As a result of these incidents, in 2007 the FDA ordered the drugs' manufacturers to issue strong new label warnings about the risks of unusual behavior and to produce brochures about safe use.

Although rare, these incidents highlight the need for people who use sleep medications to be aware of the potential side effects and to use them properly. Always allow enough time for sleep, use only as directed, and avoid alcohol. If you experience any unusual occurrences, talk to your doctor right away.

than benzodiazepines. They note that insomnia is often related to depression and antidepressants have fewer regulatory restrictions than benzodiazepines, so they're easier to prescribe. However, comparison studies have not been done. In addition to doxepin, other antidepressants commonly prescribed for insomnia include trazodone (Desyrel) and amitriptyline (Elavil, Endep).

Studies of depressed people who also have sleep problems show that these medications reduce the time it takes to fall asleep and the number of nighttime arousals. How they work isn't clear, but sleep may result from a sedative effect. In addition, the drugs' ability to ease anxiety and mild depression may make it easier for people with these problems to relax and fall asleep.

The effect of antidepressants on sleep quality varies; in general, they reduce REM sleep but have little impact on deep sleep. Side effects—namely dizziness, dry mouth, upset stomach, weight gain, and sexual dysfunction—are common. These drugs also can increase leg movements during sleep. Some people find certain antidepressants make them feel nervous or restless, so the medication can actually make insomnia worse. It's not clear if these medications lead to tolerance or rebound insomnia.

Melatonin-receptor agonist

Ramelteon (Rozerem) mimics the body's naturally produced melatonin, a hormone that promotes sleep. It stimulates the same receptors as melatonin in the suprachiasmatic nucleus, the part of the brain that controls the circadian cycle of sleep and wakefulness. Ramelteon has a more potent effect than over-the-counter melatonin, which helps some people fall asleep faster and can be used to change the circadian sleep phase. Ramelteon has a short half-life of two to five hours. Since it wears off quickly, the drug is approved to treat insomnia for people who have trouble falling asleep at bedtime rather than those who have trouble staying asleep.

Ramelteon's most common side effect is dizziness, and it may also worsen symptoms of depression. People who have severe liver damage or who use the antidepressant fluvoxamine (Luvox) shouldn't take it. Citing clinical studies that found ramelteon did not cause tolerance, dependence, or rebound insomnia, the drug's manufacturer promotes it for long-term use.

The drug may be more likely to benefit older rather than younger people, since people produce less melatonin as they age. However, older people's primary sleep problem tends to be waking up during the night, not falling asleep at the beginning of the night, suggesting ramelteon's usefulness may be limited. More studies and clinical experience should help clarify the picture.

Orexin-receptor antagonist

Suvorexant (Belsomra) works by blocking orexin (also known as hypocretin)—a neurotransmitter that promotes wakefulness. People with narcolepsy, who experience sudden "sleep attacks," lack orexin-producing cells in their brains—a discovery that led to the development of suvorexant.

Suvorexant should be taken within 30 minutes of going to bed and only if you can sleep for at least seven hours. Like some of the nonbenzodiazepines, it can cause next-day drowsiness, in addition to other side effects such as dizziness, headache, and unusual dreams. Because this medication doesn't have much of a track record (it was FDA-approved in 2014), it's too soon to know how it compares with other available options.

Over-the-counter sleep aids

Drugstores carry a bewildering variety of over-the-counter sleep products, and there's clearly a market for them. One small survey of people ages 60 and over found that more than a quarter of them had taken nonprescription sleep aids in the preceding year—and that one in 12 did so daily. But do these products work? And if you try them, should you choose a sleeping pill, an herbal remedy, or a dietary supplement?

Standard nonprescription sleeping pills

Behind the riot of competing brands, this class of products is surprisingly straightforward. Each one—whether a tablet, capsule, or gelcap—contains an antihistamine as its primary active ingredient. Most over-the-counter sleep aids—including Nytol, Sominex, and others—contain 25 to 50 milligrams (mg) of the antihistamine diphenhydramine. A few, such as Unisom SleepTabs, contain 25 mg of doxylamine, another antihistamine.

Over-the-counter antihistamines have a sedating effect and are generally safe. But they can cause nausea and, more rarely, fast or irregular heartbeat, blurred vision, or heightened sensitivity to sunlight. Complications are generally more common in children and in people over age 60. Diphenhydramine blocks the brain chemical acetylcholine, which is essential for normal brain function. A study that pooled findings from 27 studies on the effect of medications like diphenhydramine found that elderly people who took these drugs faced a higher risk of cognitive problems, including delirium. Alcohol heightens the effect of these medications, which can also interact adversely with some drugs. If you take nonprescription sleeping pills, be sure to ask your physician about the possibility of interactions with other medications.

Sleep experts generally advise against using these medications, largely because of their side effects but also because they are often ineffective. And there's no information about the safety of taking these drugs over the long term.

Dietary supplements

According to one survey, about 1.4% of adult Americans have used some form of alternative medicine (mostly herbal supplements) for insomnia or trouble sleeping.

As with other dietary supplements, the FDA does not regulate these products, so they aren't tested for safety, effectiveness, quality, or accuracy of labeling. Although marketed as "natural," these products may contain biologically active substances that can have side effects or interact with other medications or supplements. If you're thinking about using such products (or already do so), be sure to tell your doctor.

Many herbal products include a variety of active ingredients, some of which might interact unfavorably with other medications you're taking. Even a single herb is a complex chemical stew. Valerian root extract, for example, contains more than 100 specifically identified substances. Researchers don't know precisely which one of these accounts for the herb's effect, nor can they say exactly how they might interact with other medications. Finally, the per-dose price of these remedies varies far more than that of standard sleeping pills.

Scientific understanding of these substances is limited, and what we know generally comes from small, short-term studies. Thus, most doctors discourage the use of herbal medicines as sleep aids. But the market for such products is booming. Readily available alternative sleep remedies include the following.

Valerian (Valeriana officinalis). A few studies suggest that valerian is mildly sedating and can help people fall asleep and improve their sleep quality. However, a review in the *Journal of Clinical Sleep Medicine* pointed out that most of the studies were small and flawed, and that even the positive studies showed only a mild effect. The most common reported side effects are headaches, dizziness, itching, and gastrointestinal disturbances.

As with other unregulated remedies, the quality of valerian-containing products varies widely. A report by ConsumerLab—a commercial laboratory that periodically tests the quality of herbal remedies—found that nearly a quarter of valerian-based products appeared to contain no valerian whatsoever, and an equal number had less than half the amount claimed on their labels.

Chamomile. Tea made from this flower, a member of the daisy family, is a traditional remedy long used to help people relax and become drowsy. Chamomile is both mild and safe, although rare allergic reactions, including bronchial constriction, can occur. If you're allergic to plants in the daisy family, which includes ragweed, you should probably avoid this herb. There are no scientific studies showing chamomile is effective in treating insomnia.

Synthetic melatonin. The brain's production of the hormone melatonin peaks in the late evening, in conjunction with the onset of sleep. Since the 1990s, a synthetic version has been widely available in the United States as a supplement at health food stores and pharmacies. In Great Britain and Canada, melatonin is classified as a medicine and available by prescription only.

Despite some initial enthusiasm for synthetic melatonin, most subsequent research has been disappointing, finding either minimal benefits or none at all. A review of the melatonin research by the federal Agency for Healthcare Research and Quality (AHRQ) concluded that the supplement "is not effective in treating most sleep disorders." However, a subset of people do appear to benefit: those whose insomnia results from delayed sleep phase syndrome, a circadian rhythm disorder in which people don't start to feel sleepy until hours after the conventional bedtime. The AHRQ review found that melatonin enables people with this disorder to fall asleep an average of nearly 40 minutes faster than they would with a placebo.

Melatonin has a short half-life (one or two hours) and does not appear to pose any major health risks when taken for a short time. The most commonly reported side effects are nausea, headache, and dizziness. Its long-term effects are unknown. A controlled-release version with a longer duration of action, called Circadin (available in some other countries but not in the United States) may help some people with insomnia, according to European research. ▼

Breathing disorders in sleep

Although relaxed and steady breathing is natural for most sleepers, some people snore so loudly that they literally wake the neighbors. Loud snoring may be a sign of sleep apnea, a life-threatening condition marked by frequent interruptions in breathing. In most cases, however, people who snore only suffer from simple snoring produced when the muscles of the airways relax during sleep—a condition that doesn't cause medical complications but may disrupt the sleep of others nearby.

Snoring

When you fall asleep, muscles in your airway relax, causing the airway to narrow. Snoring occurs when it narrows too much, causing turbulent airflow. The surrounding tissue vibrates, producing noise. One population study reported that 24% of women and 40% of men were habitual snorers.

If your nasal passages are swollen by a cold, allergies, or a reaction to smoke, you may snore temporarily. But a number of physical characteristics can also contribute to long-term problems with snoring. These include

- a deviated septum (a misalignment of the bone and cartilage that separates the two sides of the nose)
- an elongated soft palate (the fleshy, flexible area toward the back of the roof of the mouth)
- a large uvula (the fleshy piece of tissue that hangs down from the soft palate; a normal-sized one clears the top of the tongue when the mouth is open)
- enlarged tonsils (the small masses of soft tissue on both sides of the back of the throat)

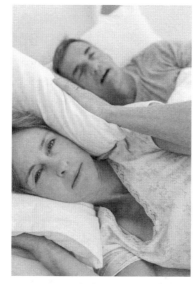

Losing even a little weight can help reduce snoring. Also quit smoking, and forgo alcohol and sleeping pills, which all contribute to the problem.

- enlarged adenoids (small lumps of tissue located above the tonsils)
- a very small jaw
- excess fat in the neck area.

The hormones progesterone and estrogen may play a protective role; before menopause, women snore less than men, but snoring increases among women later in life. Many women snore late in their pregnancies, a phenomenon attributed to hormone-related swelling of airway tissues.

Although snoring is rarely life-threatening, sleep specialists take even simple snoring seriously. A person who snores heavily deserves a thorough examination of the throat, mouth, palate, tongue, and neck and may need to undergo sleep studies.

Treatments for snoring

Hundreds of devices are marketed as aids for people who wish to stop snoring or improve their nighttime breathing. Some encourage you to sleep on your side; others are dental appliances that try to keep your airway open by preventing your tongue from falling back or by moving your jaw forward. Check with your physician before investing in such a device. He or she may be able to recommend simple, inexpensive ways to prevent snoring. For example, some people snore only when lying on their backs, so devices that encourage lying on the side are helpful (see "Positional aids," page 33). Other people keep air passages open by raising their heads with an extra pillow or by propping up the head of the bed a few inches.

Doctors usually encourage overweight snorers to lose weight. Dropping even just a little weight (5% to 10% of your body weight) can make a difference. It may also help to quit smoking, since the irritation causes swelling of airway tissues. In addition, it makes sense to forgo alcohol, sleeping pills, and tranquilizers, all of which decrease muscle tone.

If swollen nasal tissues are the problem, a humidifier or medication may reduce swelling. An operation may be necessary to correct a deviated septum or remove large tonsils and adenoids. In extreme cases, physicians may recommend more extensive surgery, similar to that used to treat sleep apnea.

Laser surgery. For this procedure, called laser-assisted uvulopalatoplasty (LAUP), a physician uses a carbon dioxide laser to shorten the uvula and to make small cuts in the soft palate on either side of the uvula. As these nicks heal, the surrounding tissue pulls tighter and stiffens. Because snoring results from the flapping of loose tissue at the back of the soft palate, it is less likely to occur when the tissue is smaller and stiffer. Afterward, people usually have a sore throat for about a week. After five weeks of healing, the treatment may be repeated if snoring persists. Three or four procedures may be needed.

While LAUP can be quite effective in stopping snoring, the technique doesn't appear to ease apnea and may not be covered by insurance. What's more, this procedure can be dangerous for people with apnea because it removes the warning signal of this breathing disorder, so be sure you have a physician rule out sleep apnea before undergoing LAUP.

Somnoplasty. Also known as radiofrequency tissue volume reduction, this procedure was first approved to treat snoring but later became an option for obstructive sleep apnea. A doctor delivers radiofrequency waves through the tips of tiny needles inserted into the obstructive tissue to shrink it. Somnoplasty takes only a few minutes to perform and doesn't cause bleeding, but it may have to be repeated to achieve results. People typically experience some swelling immediately following the procedure; over-the-counter painkillers can usually control any pain.

Palatal implants. In this procedure, also known as the Pillar procedure, a surgeon implants up to three matchstick-sized stiffening rods made of polyester into the soft palate. The rods help keep the palate from collapsing, limiting obstruction of the back of the throat when a person falls asleep. The procedure, done under local anesthesia in an office, is reversible. If it causes pain or does not work, the rods can be removed. Sometimes the rods come out on their own, without significant discomfort. They may improve symptoms, but only if your snoring results from collapse of the palate.

Sleep apnea

Sleep apnea is a serious health condition in which breathing stops or becomes shallower hundreds of times each night. In the most common form, obstructive sleep apnea, the tongue or throat tissues block the airway (see Figure 5, page 31). Central sleep apnea, in which the brain does not send messages to the muscles that control breathing, accounts for less than 5% of cases.

Untreated, sleep apnea can have devastating consequences. The relentless daytime fatigue that often results may destroy careers, break up marriages, and lead to automobile and workplace accidents. It can even be life-threatening, contributing to the development of high blood pressure, heart failure, and stroke. A *New England Journal of Medicine* study found that

---

Test for sleep apnea with STOPBANG

A "yes" answer to three or more of these questions suggests possible sleep apnea. Ask your doctor if you should have a home sleep study.

S —Snore: Have you been told that you snore?

T —Tired: Do you often feel tired during the day?

O —Obstruction: Do you know if you briefly stop breathing while asleep, or has anyone witnessed you do this?

P —Pressure: Do you have high blood pressure or take medication for high blood pressure?

B —Body mass index (BMI): Is your BMI 30 or above? (For a calculator, see www.health.harvard.edu/bmi.)

A —Age: Are you 50 or older?

N —Neck: Is your neck circumference more than 16 inches (women) or 17 inches (men)?

G —Gender: Are you male?

---

sleep apnea doubles a person's risk of suffering a stroke over a seven-year period. And sleep apnea can wreak havoc on the cardiovascular system because the heart must work harder every time the person rouses to open his or her airway (see "Heart disease," page 17).

Sleep apnea used to be considered uncommon, and it often remained undiagnosed. Physicians rarely checked for it except in the stereotypical patient—an overweight, middle-aged man who snored. But the prevalence has soared over the past two decades, at least in part because of the obesity epidemic. Still, while more than half of the estimated 25 million Americans who have sleep apnea are overweight, many are not. The disorder affects an estimated one in four adults between the ages of 30 and 70, and the incidence rises with age.

Obstructive sleep apnea

Obstructive sleep apnea (OSA) occurs when the upper airway is blocked by excess tissue, such as a large uvula, the tongue, the tonsils, fatty deposits in the airway walls, congested nasal passages, or a floppy rim at the back of the palate. People with OSA tend to have smaller airway openings than those who don't. A narrow airway makes obstruction all the more likely when airway muscles relax at the onset of sleep.

When the airway is blocked, you cannot breathe. A potentially life-threatening lack of oxygen and buildup of carbon dioxide, as well as increasing efforts to breathe, cause you to wake and gasp loudly for air until blood oxygen levels return to normal. At worst, a person with OSA cannot breathe and sleep at the same time.

Some people with OSA repeat this cycle hundreds of times a night without being fully aware of what is happening. They don't realize how little sleep they're actually getting and may routinely feel sleepy. Others wake up after bouts of apnea and have difficulty getting back to sleep. They reason that insomnia—not a breathing problem—makes them sleepy during the day. The condition can become even more perilous if a person with OSA uses substances that further relax airway muscles or suppress arousal or breathing, such as muscle relaxants, alcohol, and some sleeping pills.

Symptoms and signs of OSA are as follows:

- **Grogginess, fatigue, and sleepiness.** People with OSA are often extremely tired during the day, often nodding off when they want to stay awake.
- **Loud, disruptive snoring.** Frequent snoring that is

Figure 5: Treating apnea with CPAP

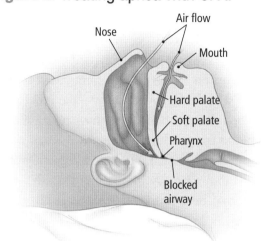

In a person with obstructive sleep apnea, the upper airway—which includes the nose, mouth, and throat—is blocked. In the example above, excess fatty tissue around the soft palate and pharynx is the culprit, but the blockage can occur anywhere along the airway. As a result, air can't enter the lungs, and the resulting drop in oxygen signals the brain to send an emergency "breathe now!" signal that briefly awakens the sleeper and makes him or her gasp for air. These pauses in breathing can last seconds to minutes and can occur up to 100 times per hour.

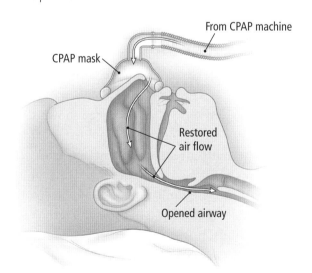

A CPAP machine delivers continuous airflow via a mask that covers the nose. The air pressure prevents the collapse of the airway when the muscles relax during sleep. This allows the person to sleep normally without interruption.

loud enough to disturb a bed partner is a hallmark of OSA. The snorer may choke, gasp, or appear to hold his or her breath during sleep.

- **Thick neck.** Men with a neck circumference of 17 inches or more and women with a neck circumference of 16 inches or more are at higher risk. As with snoring, obesity is a major risk factor, since fatty deposits surrounding the throat expand as people gain weight, narrowing the airway.
- **High blood pressure.** More than half of people with OSA have high blood pressure, caused by OSA.

OSA occurs on a spectrum. In some cases, the airway is only slightly narrowed, but people must work extra hard to inhale, although they have no significant drop in blood oxygen levels. This extra work wakes them up many times each night, and they may complain of insomnia or daytime sleepiness. The same treatments that help individuals with a fully closed airway are also effective for these cases.

Treatments for obstructive sleep apnea

Treatments for OSA fall into three general categories—lifestyle changes, devices, and surgery. Medications also may be used along with these treatments.

Lifestyle changes. Weight loss is the best treatment for weight-related OSA, but it doesn't always cure the problem. Also, because losing weight is challenging and takes a long time to achieve, most people with severe symptoms need additional treatment. Sleeping on your side instead of your back can work if you have OSA only while sleeping on your back. Everyone with OSA should avoid alcohol, sedatives, and muscle relaxants. Nasal strips, mechanical dilators, and moisturizing gels and sprays have not been shown to help.

Devices. These include the gold standard (and most commonly used) treatment for OSA, called continuous positive airway pressure; several newer treatments that are similar but less cumbersome; and dental devices that reposition the jaw and tongue.

- **Continuous positive airway pressure (CPAP).** Positive airway pressure (PAP) uses an air-pressure device connected by a hose to a mask that covers the nose. The air pressure opens the airway, preventing collapse when muscles relax during sleep. This allows you to sleep normally and breathe without interrup-

tion. With CPAP, the air pressure stays the same while you breathe in and out (see Figure 5, page 31). Many models offer options such as warmed humidified air (which alleviates nasal congestion, skin dryness, and dry mouth) and a timer that slowly builds up pressure when you turn the machine on, to give you time to adapt and fall asleep more easily. There are also a variety of mask styles, allowing you to find the one that best fits your face and is most comfortable. Most cover only the nose, but some cover both the nose and the mouth.

People usually try CPAP for the first time in a sleep laboratory, so a technician can adjust the pressure during sleep. Many people adjust to it without any problem and report that their night in the laboratory is the best night's sleep they've had in years. Others find it difficult at first to breathe out against a constant stream of air and to sleep with their mouth closed, but they usually get used to it with time.

CPAP is covered by most insurance plans. Most people procure the device on a rent-to-buy basis through their insurance companies. You can also order CPAP machines online; prices range from $500 to $1,500. CPAP generally leads to a great improvement in the amount of time spent in restorative deep sleep, which improves alertness the next day. In many cases, CPAP also reduces or eliminates high blood pressure. For some people, CPAP is a lifelong treatment.

- **BiPAP and AutoPAP.** For people who have difficulty exhaling against the pressure of CPAP, a

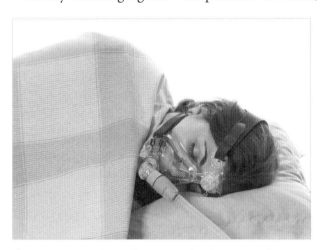

The most commonly used treatment for obstructive sleep apnea is an air-pressure device called CPAP.

refinement called bi-level PAP (often referred to by the trademarked name BiPAP) may be easier to use. It delivers air under higher pressure as you inhale and switches to a lower pressure during exhalation to make it easier for you to breathe out. AutoPAP machines take this improvement a step further by including an internal regulator that moves the pressure up and down according to required pressure needs, using the lowest level or pressure possible. While some people find these devices more comfortable, they may be more expensive.

- **Expiratory positive airway pressure.** This technology, marketed under the name Provent, relies on small, circular, single-use valves surrounded by bandage-like adhesive that you place over the opening of each nostril every night. As you breathe in, the valves open. As you breathe out, they partially close. The air that backs up in your airway as you exhale produces the positive pressure that keeps the airway open. Research suggests the device sharply cuts the number of apnea episodes a person has and eliminates OSA in about 50% of users. But not everyone finds Provent easy to use, especially people who tend to breathe through their mouth at night, or those who have nasal allergies and a stuffed-up nose. A 30-day supply of the patches costs $65 to $80 and is typically not covered by insurance. But if you can tolerate Provent, the product is far more portable than a PAP device—a special boon for frequent travelers.

- **Oral pressure therapy.** Instead of positive pressure, this therapy uses negative pressure from a small vacuum pump to open the airway. The vacuum, housed in a bedside console, is delivered through a thin tube connected to a soft, flexible mouthpiece, similar to a retainer on the teeth but that also holds the tongue in place. Early studies suggest this device—called the Winx Sleep Therapy System—may work for many people, but clinical trials are needed to determine its ultimate role in treating OSA. Although much smaller and quieter than a CPAP machine, Winx costs about the same as a high-end CPAP.

- **Dental devices.** These devices reposition the lower jaw and tongue, so that the airway remains open. They are fairly well tolerated and have a success rate of about 50% to 70% for mild to moderate OSA. One, the Mandibular Advancement Device, resembles a sports mouth guard and works by pushing the lower jaw forward and down slightly. Another, called a tongue-retaining device, holds the tongue in place to keep the airway as open as possible. These devices are less cumbersome and easier to travel with than CPAP. However, they can cause shifting of teeth and problems with the temporomandibular joint, so be sure to get the device from a dentist trained in treating people with OSA and get regular follow-ups, including a sleep study done with the device in place to make sure it eliminates the OSA.

- **Positional aids.** Some people only have apnea when they sleep on their backs, so props or devices that encourage them to sleep on their sides sometimes help. Low-tech options include wedge-shaped pillows or a tennis ball sewn into the back of a nightshirt. Another option is a device called Night Shift, which is a small monitor worn on the back of the neck. If you start sleeping on your back, it starts to vibrate with increasing intensity until you change position. It also monitors your sleep quality and how often you snore loudly, and this data can be uploaded online and shared with your doctor.

Surgery. Most surgical procedures for sleep apnea do not have good success rates. Although some people improve, a sizable percentage don't get better. And some people's symptoms actually worsen—that is, they have more episodes of apnea after the surgery than they had before.

What's behind these poor success rates? Surgeons must deal with a long soft tube of tissue that can collapse at any point—or even at several points—and

▶ Weight-loss surgery for apnea?

Bariatric surgery helps extremely obese people lose weight by reducing the size of the stomach. Initial reports suggested that the extreme weight loss following the surgery could effectively "cure" sleep apnea. But subsequent research revealed that while surgical weight loss can reduce the severity of sleep apnea and eliminate the condition in some people, others will still have sleep apnea following surgery and likely need continued treatment.

they can't always predict exactly where it might collapse in the future. Surgery corrects collapse at a single spot, so if a collapse later occurs at a different spot or in several spots, OSA can return.

That's not to say surgery is always a bad idea. If you have OSA, consult with a sleep specialist to review all your options. Then, if you decide on surgery, find a surgeon who has a lot of experience with these procedures to improve your chances for success.

Types of surgery for OSA include the following:

- **Corrective jaw surgery.** Surgery to move the upper or lower jaw forward may enlarge the upper airway for some people with OSA. Centers with specialists in this procedure report success rates up to 90%. However, the procedure requires extensive training and experience. The procedure changes the facial appearance and teeth alignment and requires an extensive recovery period.

- **Uvulopalatopharyngoplasty (UPPP).** This procedure to remove throat tissue helps about 40% to 45% of people with OSA. The rest may need to have further upper airway surgery or use PAP.

- **Upper airway stimulation therapy.** This therapy features a small device that's surgically implanted in the upper chest. The device monitors your breathing and, if needed, stimulates nerves around your tongue and airway to prevent them from collapsing. The FDA-approved system, called Inspire, reduced apnea episodes by 70% in one study.

- **Palatal implants.** Some specialists have started using palatal implants (see page 30) to treat people whose OSA results from an elongated soft palate. It's not yet clear what percentage of people benefit or how long improvements last.

- **Somnoplasty.** Originally developed to treat snoring, somnoplasty (see page 30) uses radiofrequency waves to shrink obstructive tissues when other treatments have not helped mild OSA. There are

Table 5: Medications for sleep apnea

GENERIC NAME (BRAND NAME)	SIDE EFFECTS	COMMENTS
Obstructive sleep apnea (medications are used with other therapies)		
SSRI antidepressants* fluoxetine (Prozac), paroxetine (Paxil), sertraline (Zoloft)	Upset stomach, nightmares, dry mouth, decreased sexual function	Minimally effective.
Tricyclic antidepressants* amitriptyline (Elavil), clomipramine (Anafranil), desipramine (Norpramin), imipramine (Tofranil), nortriptyline (Aventyl, Pamelor), protriptyline (Vivactil)	Blurred vision, confusion, constipation, decreased sexual function	Minimally effective.
Stimulants modafinil (Provigil), armodafinil (Nuvigil)	Headache, upset stomach, nervousness	Approved to treat residual daytime sleepiness after treatment with positive airway pressure; does not treat apnea itself.
Central sleep apnea (medications are first-line treatments)		
acetazolamide* (Diamox)	Tingling in arms and legs; nausea, vomiting, or diarrhea; changes in hearing; loss of appetite	Not to be used if allergic to sulfa drugs; not to be used in conjunction with high doses of aspirin; should not be used by people with a history of kidney stones.
oxygen	Nasal dryness and irritation	Eliminates apnea in some people; also used in obstructive sleep apnea.
theophylline* (Theo-24, Uniphyl)	Heartburn, vomiting, rash	Should be used with caution by people with a history of convulsions, heart failure, or liver disease.

Although the FDA has not approved these drugs for sleep apnea, physicians have found that they sometimes help people with this condition and therefore prescribe them.

limited data supporting its use for OSA.

Medications. Medications for OSA (see Table 5, page 34) are mainly used in conjunction with other treatments.

- **Antidepressants.** Certain classes—tricyclics and selective serotonin reuptake inhibitors (SSRIs)—slightly improve airway muscle tone. They are helpful for a small percentage of people with mild OSA.
- **Oxygen.** Supplemental oxygen, given through a tube in the nose, can prevent the drops in blood oxygen that accompany airway collapse. However, oxygen does not prevent airway collapse or sleep fragmentation, so it's used in addition to other treatments.
- **Stimulants.** Some people with OSA still feel sleepy during the day even after successful treatment. Two medications may help: modafinil (Provigil), which seems to temporarily stop the brain from making neurotransmitters that promote sleep, and a related drug, armodafinil (Nuvigil). Although both can help people with OSA who have trouble staying alert in the day, they do not address the source of the problem and should be used with other treatments, not in place of them.

Central sleep apnea

Central sleep apnea, or CSA, occurs when breathing centers in the brain fail to send the necessary messages to initiate breathing. Although the airway isn't blocked, the diaphragm and chest muscles stop moving. Shortly, falling blood oxygen and rising carbon dioxide levels set off an internal alarm, triggering the person to resume breathing (and often waking him or her as a result). This rare condition warrants a thorough evaluation to establish the underlying cause, which in turn guides treatment. CSA becomes more common as people age and is more frequent and severe in those with heart failure, chronic lung disease, or neurological damage. CSA doesn't cause snoring, but people with this problem are usually aware of waking up during the night and often complain of daytime sleepiness.

Therapy usually involves treating the underlying medical condition that has disrupted breathing. For example, if the CSA is caused by heart failure, medications to treat the heart failure may eliminate the CSA. Some people use PAP and may also receive added oxygen. For people who have CSA only as they begin to fall asleep, a mild sleeping pill may help them fall asleep and stay asleep, solving the breathing problem. Medications such as acetazolamide (Diamox) and theophylline (Theo-24, Uniphyl) benefit some people (see Table 5, page 34). ▼

Movement disorders and parasomnias

Sleep is not always as quiet and peaceful as you'd like it to be. Some people are troubled by uncontrollable leg movements, while others experience parasomnias—unusual behaviors such as walking or eating during sleep.

Movement disorders

Sleepers typically shift position every 15 to 30 minutes, and it's normal for muscles to jerk at the onset of sleep (though the cause of these twitches is a mystery). But people with certain neurological disorders may find it impossible to get a restful night's sleep.

Restless legs syndrome

Restless legs syndrome (RLS) is an exasperating condition that triggers abnormal sensations in the legs (and occasionally the arms) and an irresistible urge to move them. Moving the limbs may bring temporary relief.

RLS affects about 10% of people ages 30 to 70, two-thirds of them women. As many as half of people with RLS note that other members of the family have similar symptoms. Each child of an affected person has a 50% chance of inheriting the condition. Researchers have identified specific genes linked to the development of RLS that may account for up to half of all cases of the disorder.

Sleep deprivation is a major problem for people with RLS, as the symptoms are most prominent at night—or, in many cases, occur only at night. RLS symptoms may make it difficult to fall asleep or compel the person to get in and out of bed many times.

During the day, symptoms are worse when sitting still, and the irresistible urge to move can make it difficult for some people with RLS to take car or plane trips, enjoy a movie, or even hold a desk job. People develop a variety of coping strategies, such as pacing, doing knee bends, rocking, or stretching the leg muscles. Some people get temporary relief by rubbing

or squeezing their leg muscles, wrapping their legs in bandages, or applying cold or warm compresses. The daytime symptoms sometimes abate for a few hours, days, or even years.

Because the symptoms sound bizarre or vague—and the need to be constantly mobile seems like nervousness—people with RLS are frequently thought to have psychiatric problems. Children who have RLS are often diagnosed as having attention deficit hyperactivity disorder. Some people report that their symptoms started in adolescence and that adults attributed the problem to growing pains or back trouble.

RLS usually worsens with age (see Figure 6, below). Women may find that symptoms flare up during menstruation, pregnancy, or menopause. At least one in four pregnant women experiences restless legs.

Restless legs can be brought on by alcoholism, iron-deficiency anemia, diabetes, heart failure, or kidney failure. In some people, caffeine, stress, nicotine, fatigue, or prolonged exposure to a cold or very warm

Figure 6: Prevalence of restless legs syndrome by age

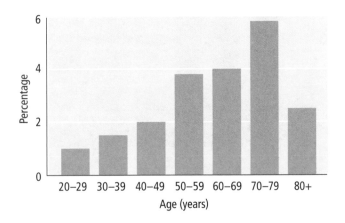

RLS can occur at any age, but it tends to be more common and severe in people over 50.

Adapted from Archives of Internal Medicine, *June 13, 2005, pp. 1286–92.*

RLS and PLMD: What's the difference?

RESTLESS LEGS SYNDROME (RLS)	PERIODIC LIMB MOVEMENT DISORDER (PLMD)
Occurs while awake, sometimes preventing sleep.	Occurs during sleep, causing partial arousals that disrupt sleep.
Involves voluntary movements—pacing, knee bends, rocking, or stretching—performed to relieve uncomfortable sensations in the lower legs and knees. Often worse after periods of inactivity and at bedtime.	Involves involuntary movements, usually repetitive flexing of the big toe, ankle, knee, and hip, typically occurring every 20 to 40 seconds. Episodes last anywhere from a few minutes to several hours.
People with RLS are aware of their symptoms, which include aching, burning, tingling, and "creepy-crawly" sensations in the legs.	Affected people usually aren't aware of their symptoms unless a bed partner complains.
Diagnosis is based on a person's description of symptoms.	Diagnosis usually requires a sleep study.

environment worsens the symptoms. Certain medications—including antihistamines, antidepressants, or lithium—can also exacerbate RLS.

Research has revealed that RLS may put a person at risk for some more significant adverse consequences in addition to the disruption of sleep. Studies have shown that the arousals caused by the leg movements are associated with increases in blood pressure and heart rate.

Periodic limb movement disorder

A neurological condition called periodic limb movement disorder (PLMD) causes people to kick and jerk their arms and legs throughout the night. Their leg and arm muscles involuntarily contract about every 20 to 40 seconds, so the movement—involving the hip, knee, or ankle—may be repeated hundreds of times a night. These so-called periodic limb movements of sleep can cause brief arousals. PLMD results when they disrupt sleep enough to produce daytime sleepiness.

Most people with RLS also have PLMD, but the reverse is not true. In fact, the two disorders have several key distinctions (see "RLS and PLMD: What's the difference?" above). The health consequences, however, may be similar.

According to some estimates, as many as 30% to 50% of people ages 65 and older have periodic limb movements of sleep. However, that figure is based on observations of leg twitches alone, and not all of these people experience the brief, unconscious awakenings that disrupt sleep.

Episodes of limb movements may last only a few minutes, or they may continue for hours, with intervals of sound sleep in between. They usually don't occur continuously throughout the night, but cluster in the first half of the night and occur mainly during non-REM sleep. Instead of proceeding smoothly through all the sleep stages in regular cycles, people with PLMD awaken for a few seconds at a time (generally without realizing it) and frequently skip back to the lighter stages of sleep. Unless a bed partner complains, people with PLMD are often oblivious to the movements and may wake up baffled at why they feel exhausted despite getting what seemed like a full night's rest.

Treatments for movement disorders

Doctors diagnose RLS and PLMD based on the individual's description of symptoms and, in some cases, observations during an overnight sleep study. Standard neurological examinations often reveal no abnormality.

Several small studies suggest that exercise can ease both RLS and PLMD; walking or other moderate exercise, such as biking or swimming, are good choices. Some people find that cold showers are beneficial, but others prefer heat. Finally, some people with mild RLS may be able to get to sleep by simply massaging their calves or stretching their legs in bed. But most people with moderate to severe RLS need medication.

Drugs that ease the tremors of Parkinson's disease also reduce the number of leg movements and thus improve quality of life for people with RLS and PLMD (see Table 6, page 38). These include bromocriptine (Parlodel), levodopa-carbidopa (Sinemet), pramipexole (Mirapex), and ropinirole (Requip). Although the drugs used to treat RLS and PLMD are the same as those used in treating Parkinson's disease, people with these sleep disorders are no more likely to develop Parkinson's disease than other individuals. In 2012, the FDA approved rotigotine (Neupro), a skin patch that delivers a long-acting, once-daily dose of medication

Table 6: Medications for movement disorders

GENERIC NAME (BRAND NAME)	SIDE EFFECTS	COMMENTS
Benzodiazepines		
clonazepam (Klonopin) temazepam (Restoril)	Clumsiness or unsteadiness, dizziness, lightheadedness, daytime drowsiness, headache	Should be used with caution by people with sleep apnea or other breathing difficulties; not to be used with alcohol or other depressants; habit-forming; withdrawal symptoms may occur if stopped abruptly.
Dopamine agents		
bromocriptine (Parlodel) levodopa-carbidopa (Sinemet) pramipexole* (Mirapex) ropinirole* (Requip) rotigotine (Neupro transdermal patch)	Abnormal movements, depression, mental changes, nausea, dizziness	Certain drugs in this class should not be used by people who are sensitive to ergot drugs, who have high blood pressure, who take monoamine oxidase inhibitors (MAOIs), or who have glaucoma. The Neupro patch may cause rash, redness, swelling, or itching.
Opiates		
oxycodone (OxyContin) oxycodone with acetaminophen (Percocet)	Depressed breathing and circulation, dizziness or lightheadedness, next-day sedation, constipation, nausea, vomiting	Risk of addiction; not to be used by people with sleep apnea; should not be used with alcohol or other depressants.
Anticonvulsants		
carbamazepine (Tegretol) gabapentin (Neurontin) gabapentin enacarbil* (Horizant) pregabalin (Lyrica) valproic acid (Depakene)	Unsteadiness, vision problems, body aches, congestion	Tegretol may reduce the number of blood cells produced by your body.

Pramipexole, ropinirole, and gabapentin enacarbil are FDA-approved to treat RLS. Other medications in this chart are not approved to treat RLS or PLMD, but physicians have found that they can help people with these conditions.

to ease restless legs syndrome. Unlike the pills, the medication doesn't go through your digestive system, so you don't have to schedule the drug around meals.

People with mild movement disorders may be prescribed clonazepam (Klonopin) or temazepam (Restoril), which may help them stay asleep during leg movements. Most people who take these medications for insomnia develop a tolerance to them after a few weeks, but this doesn't seem to happen when such drugs are taken for RLS. Antiseizure medications such as gabapentin (Neurontin), which are used to treat epilepsy, are also prescribed for RLS. A related medication called Horizant contains gabapentin enacarbil, a long-acting version of gabapentin. Opiates (opium-derived drugs) such as oxycodone (OxyContin) may be used to treat people with severe RLS symptoms who don't respond to other treatments. Opiates decrease the discomfort of RLS and, for some, dramatically reduce leg movements at night. But because of the potential for addiction, most physicians are reluctant to treat sleep disturbances with these drugs. However, when properly used, they may provide long-term benefit with little risk of addiction.

Parasomnias

Parasomnias are strange behaviors that people engage in during sleep. People with parasomnias may wake up enough to carry out complex actions, but not enough to realize what they are doing. These sleep-disrupting phenomena include sleepwalking, sleep eating, and sleep terrors.

Somnambulism and somniloquy

Somnambulism, or sleepwalking, occurs during partial awakening from deep sleep. The person's eyes are open but have a confused, glassy appearance. Sometimes sleepwalkers do strange things, such as urinate in a trash can or move furniture. Or they may simply pace or perform repetitive behaviors, such as getting dressed and undressed multiple times. They can be difficult to awaken and typically have no memory of the episode in the morning. There have been reports of somnambulists committing murder, although this is extremely rare. Episodes of sleepwalking are usually brief and benign, with few people endangering themselves or others. Scientists used to believe that sleepwalkers were acting out their dreams, but experts have determined that sleepwalking does not occur during dreaming.

Sleepwalking is common in children, probably because their brains have not yet mastered regulation of sleep and waking. The tendency seems to be inherited. Although people are more likely to sleepwalk when they're anxious or fatigued, there is little correlation between somnambulism and psychological problems. If the condition continues beyond puberty, the individual should be evaluated to determine whether sleepwalking is the result of nighttime epilepsy or a reaction to medication, extreme stress, or another sleep disorder. If the condition presents a risk of injury, a doctor may prescribe medications such as benzodiazepines.

Somniloquy, or talking in one's sleep, is nothing to worry about. People are more likely to talk in their sleep during times of stress or illness. Talking can occur during any or all stages of sleep. When awakened, people who talk in their sleep rarely remember what they said. Only occasionally can someone who talks in his or her sleep hear and respond to what someone else says.

Nocturnal eating disorders

There are two distinct nighttime eating disorders.

Nocturnal eating syndrome occurs most commonly in people with daytime eating disorders or depression. They are usually light sleepers and wake frequently. Within minutes after getting out of bed, people with this condition raid the refrigerator and begin wolfing down food. Although they aren't really hungry, they can't go back to sleep without eating. In some people with this disorder, overeating occurs only during sleep hours, not during the daytime. The person is awake and fully alert during the episode and can recall it the next day. Nocturnal eating syndrome should be treated as an eating disorder.

Sleep-related eating disorder is a combination of a sleep disorder and an eating disorder. People with this disorder experience partial arousals similar to sleepwalking, but respond by eating. Often they consume unhealthful, high-calorie food, such as cookie dough. They report being half-awake or asleep during the episodes and have very poor memory of the events or no recollection at all. Sleep-related eating disorder occurs more frequently in people with eating disorders and depression. Treatment should address both the sleep disorder and the eating disorder.

Sleep-related eating disorder occurs in children and adults and sometimes can be traced to an illness or traumatic event. A medical evaluation may reveal an ulcer, a history of strict dieting, bulimia, or a sleep problem such as narcolepsy, sleepwalking, sleep apnea, or periodic limb movement disorder. Sometimes medications prescribed for depression or insomnia can cause this disorder. A number of medicines have been tried to treat these disorders, including dopaminergic agents, anticonvulsants, antidepressants, and opiates, but results have been mixed.

Bedwetting

Bedwetting, known medically as sleep enuresis, is common among young children. It's considered a problem if it's still occurring by age six. Statistically, 80% to 85% of children are consistently dry throughout the night by age 5. After that, the number of children who continue to wet the bed decreases by about 15% per year, even without treatment, and only 1% to 2% of children still wet the bed by the time they're 15. Almost all bedwetting children eventually stay dry at night.

Bedwetting, which occurs more frequently among boys than girls, usually stems from a bladder that's not yet fully matured. Occasionally, psychological stress is to blame. Children with specific physical problems (such as a structural abnormality of the urinary tract, diabetes, or a urinary tract infection) may also have difficulty with daytime bladder control. It's important for adults to understand that, initially, children have little control over bedwetting. Punishments won't solve the problem. If your child wets the bed, stay calm as you change the child's pajamas and bed sheets and don't show disgust or disappointment.

Reminding the child to urinate before going to bed and limiting liquids in the last two hours before bedtime may reduce or eliminate the problem. Other options include setting up a token-and-reward system to motivate the child. Consult your pediatrician for further details.

Bedwetting occurs in a very small percentage of adults and is often due to an underlying medical problem or excessive caffeine or beer consumption. In men, an enlarged prostate gland that presses against the bladder may be to blame. Bedwetting may be a side effect of diuretic pills or a sign of diabetes, a bladder or kidney problem, epilepsy, or serious obstructive sleep apnea. Treatment for adult bedwetting depends on the cause.

REM sleep behavior disorder

Most people make subtle twitching movements during REM sleep, but occasionally sleepers shout, punch, or otherwise act out their dreams. This phenomenon—known as REM sleep behavior disorder—was identified in the 1980s. It's estimated to occur in one in 200 people (0.5%), and nine out of 10 people who have it are men. The disorder nearly always arises after age 50, but there are occasional reports of it occurring in younger adults and children. Approximately 70% of people with REM sleep behavior disorder go on to develop Parkinson's disease, suggesting that similar brain structures are involved in both conditions.

If the person is at risk of harming himself or others or is having daytime sleepiness from the sleep disruption, a medium-acting benzodiazepine may help suppress symptoms. Until the problem is under control, people can protect themselves and loved ones by sleeping in a separate room and putting sharp or breakable objects out of reach.

Nightmares, sleep terrors, and panic attacks

Nightmares, sleep terrors, and sleep-related panic attacks can interrupt sleep.

Nightmares. Nightmares, which usually occur early in the morning, are bad dreams that become so threatening that a person wakes in a state of fear and agitation. Nightmares occur mainly during REM sleep, when the body barely moves.

Nightmares can be a side effect of certain medications, such as antidepressants, narcotics, cholesterol-lowering statins, and barbiturates. Nightmares can also occur when a person stops taking drugs that temporarily reduce REM sleep, such as benzodiazepines. Alcoholics who stop drinking often experience dream disturbances and nightmares.

If you experience frequent nightmares that aren't linked to medication or substance use, counseling may help. The most common approach is a type of behavioral therapy known as desensitization, in which the sufferer recalls the details of the nightmare and uses relaxation techniques to overcome fear.

Sleep terrors. A sleep terror can be quite dramatic to witness. The sleeper may let out a bloodcurdling scream, sit bolt upright, and attempt to fight or flee. During an episode, which may last as long as 15 minutes, a person may seem confused and agitated. After the spell is over, he or she is likely to go right back to sleep and later may not remember what happened. For that reason, the episodes are usually more frightening to the parent or other observer than the person having the night terror. It is best to wait for the episode to resolve rather than trying to intervene or wake the sleeper. Make sure the person is safe and not likely to hurt himself or herself by moving about.

Unlike nightmares, sleep terrors occur during non-REM sleep, usually in the first hour or so after going to bed. They appear to run in families and occur most often in children. Adults with sleep terrors tend to be more agitated, anxious, and aggressive than children who have this problem. When the episodes involve violent or injurious behavior, medical treatment may be recommended. Some doctors prescribe medications such as benzodiazepines that suppress deep sleep. Hypnosis or a relaxation technique known as guided imagery may also be helpful.

Sleep-related panic attacks. People may awaken suddenly because of episodes of intense panic characterized by a racing heartbeat, sweating, trembling, breathlessness, or the feeling that they may be dying. Anti-anxiety drugs are often useful for these attacks. ◆

Narcolepsy

Narcolepsy is a disorder affecting the regulation of the sleep/wake cycle. People with narcolepsy experience bouts of extreme daytime sleepiness and tend to fall asleep suddenly at inappropriate times. These "sleep attacks" seem to arise from an abrupt switch from wakefulness into REM sleep. The brain somehow skips the normal progression of sleep stages, entering into a dreamlike state immediately after a person lies down to sleep—or in the middle of daytime activities, such as talking, eating, or driving. Sudden muscle weakness (known medically as cataplexy) may also occur, causing a person to suddenly go limp or to fall.

The disorder affects about one in 2,000 people and usually appears between ages 15 to 30. It affects men and women equally and has a genetic component: having a close relative makes a person 20 to 40 times more likely to have it. On average, it takes five years of symptoms and visits to five physicians before a diagnosis of narcolepsy is made. This is because sleepiness may be the only symptom. If cataplexy occurs, it may be misdiagnosed as epilepsy or fainting.

In the late 1990s, researchers discovered that many cases of narcolepsy result from the lack of a brain chemical called hypocretin (also called orexin) that normally maintains wakefulness and helps regulate sleep. People with narcolepsy lose the cells that make hypocretin. The discovery of the gene that makes hypocretin and the location of its production in the brain has spurred research into new ways to diagnose and treat this disorder. Researchers have also found a link between narcolepsy and variations in a gene that controls immune function. They speculated that the loss of hypocretin-producing cells may stem from an autoimmune process, in which the body attacks itself.

Symptoms of narcolepsy

All people with narcolepsy are excessively sleepy and struggle to stay awake during the day, which often causes them to have great trouble completing tasks. In addition, they may have a number of other symptoms, most of which are manifestations of the REM sleep stage occurring during wakefulness. Most people have more than one but only rarely have all of the following additional symptoms.

Sleep attacks. A person may suddenly fall asleep for a few seconds to several minutes when relaxing or even while carrying on a conversation. These attacks may be more frequent when a person is doing something monotonous or repetitive. If REM sleep and dreaming occur immediately, the person sometimes makes conversation that is appropriate to the dream instead of the actual situation.

Cataplexy. A person may suddenly lose muscle tone while awake, causing the head to fall forward and the knees to buckle. Most attacks last for less than 30 seconds and may go unnoticed, but in severe cases, the person may fall and stay paralyzed for as long as several minutes. Laughter, anger, or other strong emotions often trigger cataplexy, which occurs when the brain mechanism that paralyzes muscles during REM sleep becomes activated.

Sleep paralysis. A terrifying feeling of paralysis may occur during the transition between wakefulness and sleep if the REM stage begins before a person is fully asleep. Although muscle control usually returns within a few minutes, episodes can cause great anxiety.

Hypnagogic hallucinations. When REM dreaming occurs during wakefulness, the vivid and often frightening images, known as hypnagogic hallucinations, are difficult to distinguish from reality. A person may see prowlers or believe that his or her house is on fire. This usually happens just at sleep onset or upon awakening. This condition can be confused with mental illness because its symptoms resemble those of some psychotic disorders.

Disturbed nighttime sleep. Just as sleep intrudes during the day, unwelcome awakenings can occur at night, depriving people with narcolepsy of restorative rest and worsening their daytime drowsiness. Some feel as if they have hardly slept at all.

Automatic behavior. Because of their profound exhaustion, people with narcolepsy perform many routine tasks without being fully aware of what they are doing. For example, one man washed and dried the dishes and then stacked them in the refrigerator, but he had no recollection of doing so.

Diagnosing narcolepsy

Doctors suspect narcolepsy in people who are excessively sleepy with no other apparent cause, especially if the person also develops one of the other symptoms. Confirming the diagnosis requires an overnight and daytime sleep study. On the overnight study, the person typically falls asleep quickly, goes into REM sleep much faster than usual, and has no other sleep disorder that could cause sleepiness. The next day, the person undergoes a multiple sleep latency test: a series of five nap opportunities, spaced at two-hour intervals throughout the day. A person with narcolepsy falls asleep very quickly and quickly enters REM sleep. Rested people without narcolepsy take longer to fall asleep during the naps or don't sleep at all. If they do sleep, they don't enter REM sleep in the short, 20-minute sleep period permitted during the test.

Treatments for narcolepsy

Treatment for narcolepsy is geared toward improving wakefulness during the day and preventing REM-related symptoms.

The first-line drugs are two "wakefulness-promoting agents," modafinil (Provigil) and armodafinil (Nuvigil), which are taken once a day in the morning. Exactly how these medications work isn't clear, but they appear to boost levels of the neurotransmit-

Table 7: Medications for narcolepsy

GENERIC NAME (BRAND NAME)	USE	SIDE EFFECTS, COMMENTS
Stimulants		
dextroamphetamine (Dexedrine, Adderall) methylphenidate (Ritalin, Metadate, Concerta, others)	To counter daytime sleepiness	Nervousness, insomnia, loss of appetite, nausea, dizziness, irregular heartbeat, headaches, changes in blood pressure and pulse, weight loss. Potential for abuse. Should not be used by people who take monoamine oxidase inhibitors (MAOIs) or who have glaucoma.
armodafinil* (Nuvigil) modafinil* (Provigil)	To counter daytime sleepiness	Anxiety, headache, nausea, nervousness, insomnia. Less potential for abuse than other stimulants.
Tricyclic antidepressants		
clomipramine (Anafranil) desipramine (Norpramin) imipramine (Tofranil) protriptyline (Vivactil)	To prevent cataplexy and other REM-related symptoms	Dizziness, dry mouth, blurred vision, weight gain, constipation, trouble urinating, drowsiness, disturbance of heart rhythm. Should not be used with MAOIs or during immediate recovery from heart attack.
SSRI antidepressants		
fluoxetine (Prozac) paroxetine (Paxil) sertraline (Zoloft)	To prevent cataplexy and other REM-related symptoms	Nausea, dry mouth, headache, loss of appetite, nervousness, diarrhea or constipation, sweating, and sexual problems. Should not be used with MAOIs.
Anticataplectic		
sodium oxybate* (Xyrem)	To prevent cataplexy, improve nighttime sleep, and reduce daytime sleepiness	Abdominal pain, chills, dizziness, abnormal dreams, drowsiness, stomach discomfort. Must be taken at bedtime and again during the middle of the night. Potential for abuse.

*Armodafinil, modafinil, and sodium oxybate are FDA-approved to treat narcolepsy symptoms. Other medications in this table are not, but physicians have found they often help people with narcolepsy and therefore prescribe them.

ter dopamine. Older drugs, including methylphenidate (Ritalin) or dextroamphetamine (Dexedrine) are less commonly prescribed because of their side effects, which include high blood pressure, anorexia (extreme weight loss), and addiction (see Table 7, page 42). Even with medications, however, people are never as alert as they would be if they didn't have narcolepsy.

In most people, antidepressants that suppress REM sleep—such as fluoxetine (Prozac), sertraline (Zoloft), paroxetine (Paxil), clomipramine (Anafranil), or venlafaxine (Effexor)—can also prevent cataplexy and other REM-related symptoms.

Another medication for cataplexy is sodium oxybate (Xyrem), also known as gamma hydroxybutyrate (GHB). This medication helps decrease the number of cataplexy episodes and may improve nighttime sleep and reduce daytime sleepiness as well. Because of its chemical properties, it must be taken at bedtime and again during the middle of the night. Xyrem is tightly regulated because of its potential for misuse; it has been associated with criminal acts such as date rape. ▼

Disturbances of sleep timing

If your internal clock is out of sync with the usual day/night, wake/sleep pattern, you may long for sleep when you need to be awake—or stay up until the wee hours of the morning without feeling tired.

Delayed sleep phase syndrome

Almost everyone is programmed for a day that lasts slightly longer than 24 hours, but light and other cues keep their sleep/wake cycles in sync with the usual 24-hour schedule. By contrast, "night owls" are less sensitive to these cues. Left to their own devices, they would generally go to sleep and wake up much later than other people each day. Only by relying on external strategies and devices, such as alarm clocks, do they manage to stay in sync with a more conventional schedule. Night owls typically have trouble getting much done in the morning.

If you're a night owl, you may be able to synchronize your schedule with others by going to bed and getting up at the same time every day. However, it's easy for your sleep patterns to go awry when you go on vacation or retire. Night owls often find that a minor shift in sleep/wake cycles—such as the onset of daylight savings time, a coast-to-coast trip, or a weekend of late-night parties—can throw them off kilter unless they force themselves to stick to a schedule.

Resetting your internal clock

Exposure to bright light as directed by a sleep specialist—a technique known as light therapy—may be useful in treating delayed sleep phase syndrome. Upon awakening, you typically sit for 30 minutes facing a specially manufactured box that emits bright light with a minimal amount of ultraviolet light. Initial studies used white light, which contains the entire spectrum of light wavelengths. Later studies have suggested that blue light is the most potent part of the spectrum for resetting the circadian clock.

Another option is to move your bedtime progressively later until you've shifted around the clock and are back in sync. To do this, go to bed three hours later each night. Once you have synchronized your schedule to match that of the other people around you, wake yourself up at the same time each day.

A delayed sleep phase can also be reset in a single weekend. This requires staying up all night on Friday and all day Saturday, then going to bed around 10 p.m. On Sunday, get up at 7 a.m. From then on, adhere closely to the same bedtime and waking time seven days a week.

Yet another option for treating delayed sleep phase syndrome is to take 1 to 3 milligrams of melatonin at your desired bedtime, which may help reset your sleep schedule.

Advanced sleep phase syndrome

People whose body rhythm cycles are shifted much earlier go to bed earlier, wake up in the early morning, and eventually can't stay awake past early evening. This condition, called advanced sleep phase syndrome, is more common among older people. Treatments being studied include bright light therapy in the evening, which helps reset the body's clock, and carefully timed doses of melatonin.

Non-24-hour sleep/wake rhythm disorder

This unusual circadian rhythm disorder is marked by the continual shifting of the circadian sleep phase later each day, so that people get sleepy at different times each day. This problem is most commonly seen in blind individuals who are not sensitive to the "clock-setting" effects of light. This can be a debilitating condition for some people, creating problems with maintaining a job or desired social life because

Ways to avoid jet lag

There are two basic strategies. On a brief trip just one or two time zones away, it may be possible to wake up, eat, and sleep on home time. Schedule appointments for times when you would be alert at home.

On longer trips, to help you adjust to the new time zone, try the following.

- **Gradually switch before the trip.** For several days before you leave, move mealtimes and bedtime incrementally closer to the schedule of your destination (see Figure 7, at right). Even a partial switch may help.

- **During the flight, drink plenty of fluids, but not caffeine or alcohol.** Caffeine and alcohol promote dehydration, which worsens the symptoms of jet lag. They can also disturb sleep.

- **Switch your bedtime as rapidly as possible upon arrival.** Don't turn in until it's bedtime in the new time zone.

- **Use the sun to help you readjust.** If you need to wake up earlier in the new setting (you've flown west to east), get out in the early morning sun. If you need to wake up later (you've flown east to west), expose yourself to late afternoon sunlight.

Figure 7: Reset your biological clock

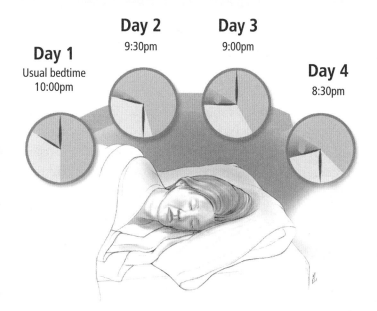

Day 1 Usual bedtime 10:00pm
Day 2 9:30pm
Day 3 9:00pm
Day 4 8:30pm

Here's one way to help reset your biological clock when you travel through time zones. If you'll be traveling through several time zones, as when flying coast to coast, you can gradually adjust your sleep time. For example, three days before you plan to travel from the West Coast to the East Coast, go to bed half an hour earlier than usual, and get up half an hour earlier the next morning. The next night, go to bed an hour earlier than usual and get up an hour earlier. The day before you travel, make it 90 minutes. By the fourth day—the day of your trip—you'll find it easier to adjust to your new time zone.

of the continual mismatch of schedules and internal rhythms. Recently, a new melatonin-receptor agonist, tasimelteon (Hetlioz), has been approved for use in blind individuals with this condition.

Jet lag

Many people find that crossing several time zones makes their internal clocks go haywire. In addition to having headaches, stomach upset, and difficulty concentrating, they may suffer from fitful sleep.

Younger people usually adapt more quickly to time changes than older people. It takes about a day to adjust for every time zone crossed. Most people have more difficulty traveling eastward, but older people may have more symptoms traveling westward.

The standard way to handle jet lag is to try to sleep only at night upon arrival and to get up early in the morning, although it may be difficult the first few days. You can also gradually adjust your sleep time prior to leaving (see Figure 7, above). This way your body can start adjusting to the new time zone as soon as possible. Short-term use of timed doses of melatonin or ramelteon to shift circadian rhythms or over-the-counter or prescription sleep aids to help you sleep at night also can be helpful.

Sunday insomnia

Some people have trouble falling asleep on Sunday nights. Anxiety about work or school on Monday may play a role, but often, the most important factor is weekend changes in sleep habits. When you stay up late Friday night and sleep in Saturday morning, you are primed to stay up even later Saturday night and sleep in the next day. By Sunday evening, your body's clock is programmed to stay up late, so it's hard to get to sleep on time. People with Sunday insomnia may feel their anxiety mount as they anticipate a difficult night ahead.

The best way to avoid this Sunday insomnia is to maintain the same wake-up time and bedtime on the weekends as during weekdays. If this isn't possible and you end up staying up later than usual on Friday and Saturday, the next best thing is to force yourself to get up at your weekday wake-up time and take an early afternoon nap on Saturday and Sunday. This way, you maintain the same wake-up time but still compensate for your sleep deprivation.

Shift work

More than 20% of American workers—including health care workers, police officers, security guards, and transit workers—are on the evening or night shift. About 60% to 70% of shift workers experience sleep disturbances. These people fall asleep on the job two to five times more often than day-shift workers do. Sleepiness can be catastrophic for people in these vital roles. Sleep-deprived physicians, for example, make a greater number of errors than their better-rested colleagues. Fatigue often plays a role in overnight rail, plane, truck, and maritime accidents.

Shift workers' sleep disruption can be eased somewhat by incorporating scheduled breaks, by rotating shifts from day to evening to night rather than the other way around, or by maintaining the same schedule seven days a week. Shift workers can also benefit from practicing good sleep hygiene (see "Practical tips for sounder sleep," page 13). Dark curtains or eyeshades can keep daylight out, and running a fan can help block external noise.

Shift workers need to enlist the help of family members to get enough sleep while maintaining a schedule at odds with the rest of the world. The most successful shift workers are those who block out time for sleep in advance and then are vigilant about protecting their sleep time from outside intrusions. Light therapy is sometimes recommended to help people get used to a new schedule, as is the short-term use of sleep medications.

Seasonal affective disorder

In most of North America, winter means less exposure to sunlight. As the days get shorter, some people find themselves depressed, sleepy, and drawn to high-carbohydrate foods.

Researchers speculate that people who suffer from this condition, called seasonal affective disorder (SAD), produce too much melatonin (or are extra-sensitive to normal amounts of this drowsiness-inducing hormone) and don't make enough serotonin, which may encourage carbohydrate cravings. Exposure to bright light in the morning for 30 minutes may alleviate the symptoms of SAD and help people wake up in the mornings. Antidepressants can also be helpful. ◗

Evaluation of sleep disturbances

Surveys suggest that although two-thirds of Americans have sleep problems at some time in their lives, most of them suffer in silence. They enjoy life less, are less productive, and endure more illnesses and accidents at home, on the job, and on the road.

When to seek help

The American Academy of Sleep Medicine recommends seeking medical advice if sleep deprivation has compromised your daytime functioning for more than a month. Don't hesitate to ask for help when you're sleeping badly following a death in the family or other stressful event. A physician may suggest the short-term use of a sedative to help you sleep at night. This may help you cope better during the day and prevent the development of a long-term sleep disorder.

It's not always easy for people to get an evaluation and treatment for a sleep problem. Doctors trained in the United States receive roughly three hours of instruction on this topic during four years of medical school. According to a National Sleep Foundation survey, most primary care physicians do not routinely ask their patients about sleep. And while most of the physicians who took part in the survey admitted they had limited knowledge about sleep-related matters, more than half did not consult with an expert in sleep medicine. So it's in your best interest to seek out the help you need.

Your sleep history

A sleep disturbance cannot be accurately diagnosed unless your physician is familiar with your sleep habits and history. This information may be gleaned from an interview or from written questionnaires that you review and discuss with your doctor (see "A sample sleep history questionnaire," page 49, and "Test for sleep apnea with STOPBANG," page 30). A bedroom

---

How sleepy are you?

Sleep specialists often use this measure, called the Epworth Sleepiness Scale, to gauge a person's level of daytime sleepiness. Imagine yourself in the following situations, and then select your likelihood of dozing using the 0–3 scale below. Add up these numbers. If you score 10 points or more, consider seeing a physician for an evaluation.

Scale: 0 = would never doze
1 = slight chance of dozing
2 = moderate chance of dozing
3 = high chance of dozing

SITUATION	SCORE
Sitting and reading	
Watching TV	
Sitting inactive in a public place, like a theater or meeting	
As a passenger in a car for an hour without a break	
Lying down to rest in the afternoon	
Sitting and talking to someone	
Sitting quietly after lunch (when you've had no alcohol)	
In a car while stopped in traffic	
TOTAL	

---

partner may be able to help answer some of these questions and should contribute to the discussion.

Some people are so used to sleep deprivation that they don't realize they're tired; instead, they may see themselves as lazy, lethargic, or not very motivated. Or they may not think it is unusual to fall asleep at a movie or while sitting at dinner with friends. Someone considered by family members to be a "good napper," able to drop off quickly and sleep through anything, may actually be displaying signs of abnormal sleepiness. Your physician may ask how likely you are to doze off in certain situations. The less appropriate the circumstances (such as waiting in traffic while driv-

Discovering the cause of sleeplessness

Depression and anxiety can both disrupt sleep. To gauge whether either one is causing your sleep problem, answer the questions below.

ARE YOU DEPRESSED?	YES	NO
1. I feel downhearted, blue, and sad.		
2. I don't enjoy the things I used to.		
3. I have felt so low I've thought of suicide.		
4. I feel that I'm not useful or needed.		
5. I notice that I'm losing/gaining weight.		
6. I have trouble sleeping through the night.		
7. I am restless and can't keep still.		
8. My mind isn't as clear as it used to be.		
9. I get tired for no reason.		
10. I feel hopeless about the future.		

You may be suffering from depression if you checked yes for at least five of these statements (at least one of which must be either number 1 or number 2) and if these symptoms have persisted for at least two weeks. Seek professional help immediately if you checked yes for number 3.

ARE YOU ANXIOUS?*	YES	NO
1. Do you feel upset or tense, maybe without even knowing why?		
2. Does your heart often race uncontrollably?		
3. Are your hands often sweaty, clammy, or extremely cold?		
4. Do you often have a lump in your throat?		
5. Do you have difficulty slowing down or relaxing?		
6. Do you often feel insecure or anxious?		
7. Do you often feel ill at ease?		
8. Do you often feel tired without any reason?		
9. Do you often worry about things you've said that might have hurt somebody's feelings?		
10. Do you tend to worry, even over things that you realize don't matter?		
11. Are you presently worrying over a possible misfortune?		
12. Do you often feel nervous, jittery, or high-strung?		
13. Are you more apprehensive about the future than other people are?		

If you answered yes to three of these questions, anxiety may be causing your sleep problems. If you answered yes to five or more, you may need to seek professional help.

Reprinted with permission from No More Sleepless Nights by Peter Hauri, Ph.D., and Shirley Linde, Ph.D.

ing or having a conversation), the more dangerously sleepy you are considered to be (see "How sleepy are you?" on page 47).

The psychiatric interview

Sleep disturbances, particularly insomnia, are often related to psychological difficulties that respond well to treatment once they've been identified. Physicians may screen problem sleepers for symptoms of depression, anxiety, childhood physical or sexual abuse, or other psychological problems or traumatic experiences (see "Discovering the cause of sleeplessness," at left). If one of these conditions is diagnosed, your primary care physician may refer you to a psychologist or psychiatrist for treatment.

Sleep testing

Most people with sleep problems don't need to visit a sleep laboratory. Insomnia and circadian rhythm disorders, for example, can be diagnosed in the doctor's office based on a thorough history and physical examination. However, when a doctor suspects a sleep disorder such as narcolepsy, periodic limb movement disorder, sleep apnea, or one of the parasomnias, he or she may recommend formal sleep testing, which can be done in a sleep laboratory or with portable devices you can use at home.

Fees depend on the level of testing required. Some people require a one-time consultation with a sleep specialist, which may run a few hundred dollars. Staying overnight in a sleep laboratory costs between $800 and $1,500. Home tests can cost from $300 to $600. Check with your insurance company in advance because reimbursement varies and may depend on your diagnosis.

The American Academy of Sleep Medicine has a listing of more than 2,500 accredited sleep disorders centers and more than 5,600 board-certified sleep specialists (see "Resources," page 52). Some centers allow you to make an appointment directly, while others require a physician referral. The center will request medical records and may send you a sleep questionnaire or diary to use before your visit. You may also be asked to change your sleep habits in certain ways

A sample sleep history questionnaire

Your physician may ask you some of the following questions during an evaluation for a sleep problem. You may find it helpful to write down your answers to these questions and bring the completed questionnaire to the exam so you and your doctor can discuss it.

What bothers you most about your sleep habits?

_____

_____

How long have you had trouble sleeping, and what do you think started the problem? Did it come on suddenly?

_____

_____

How would you describe your usual night's sleep?

_____

_____

What time do you go to bed, and when do you wake up?

_____

_____

How long does it take you to fall asleep?

_____

Once you're asleep, do you sleep through the night or wake up frequently?

_____

_____

What's your bedroom like?

_____

_____

What do you do in the few hours before bedtime?

_____

_____

Do you follow the same sleep pattern during the week and on weekends? If not, how are weekends different?

_____

_____

How well do you sleep on the first few nights when you're away from home? At home, do you sleep better in your bedroom or in another room in the house?

_____

_____

Do you often feel sleepy during the day?

_____

Do you fall asleep at inappropriate times or places?

_____

Do allergies or nasal congestion bother you at night?

_____

Have you ever been in a car accident or had a close call because you nodded off at the wheel?

_____

_____

Do you have physical aches and pains that interfere with sleep?

_____

_____

What medications or drugs (including alcohol and nicotine) do you use? Have you ever taken sleep medications? If so, which ones?

_____

_____

Do you often have indigestion at night?

_____

Do you ever feel discomfort or a fidgety sensation in your legs and feet when you lie down? Do you have to get up and walk around to relieve the feeling?

_____

_____

Do you kick or thrash around at night?

_____

Do you ever have trouble breathing when you lie down, or do you awaken because it's hard to breathe?

_____

Does your bed partner or roommate mention that you snore loudly or gasp for air at night?

_____

_____

Do you ever awaken with a choking sensation or a sour taste in your mouth?

_____

_____

Do you wake up with a headache or with cramps in your legs?

_____

_____

How have you been feeling emotionally? Does your life seem to be going as well as you would like?

_____

_____

before scheduling the visit. Sometimes these changes alone correct the problem.

Laboratory sleep tests

These tests provide the most reliable way of diagnosing sleep fragmentation disorders such as obstructive sleep apnea, periodic limb movement disorder, or seizure disorders and determining their severity. When you spend the night in a sleep laboratory, you'll wear your own nightclothes and you can use a pillow from home. You can take your regular medications, but the clinicians will need to know what they are. The lab usually provides a regular bed in a private room with a bathroom attached. The room is kept as quiet as possible.

After a technician sets up the sleep-monitoring equipment, you'll be left alone to relax until bedtime. Throughout the night, laboratory staff will monitor the instruments in a nearby control room. Procedures used may include polysomnography, audio and video recording, and daytime sleep tests.

Polysomnography. In this procedure, small wafer-thin electrodes and other sensors are pasted on specific body sites to take a variety of readings during the night. They may be placed on your scalp to track brain waves; under your chin to measure fluctuations in muscle tension (called an electromyogram, or EMG); near your eyes to measure eye movements; near your nostrils to measure airflow; on your earlobe or finger to measure the amount of oxygen in your blood (using a device called an oximeter); on your chest or back to record heart rate and rhythm; on your legs to record twitches or jerks; and over your rib muscles or around the rib cage and abdomen to monitor breathing.

Readings are collected on a single printout (called a polysomnogram) and analyzed by a technician and physician. If a breathing problem is detected early on, you may be awakened and given treatment, such as PAP, during the second half of the night. This allows the sleep experts to monitor how well the treatment works for you. Sometimes this process requires two nights. A standard polysomnogram cannot diagnose sleep-related epilepsy. If your doctor suspects that you have a seizure disorder, you may also undergo a full electroencephalogram (EEG) during the night.

Audio and video recording. Audio equipment may be used to record snoring, talking during sleep, or other sounds. A video may also be taken to compare with the polysomnogram. This may show, for example, that you snore only when in a certain position. Signs of movement disorders (such as periodic limb movement disorder) or parasomnias will probably be apparent on the video.

Daytime sleep tests. After a night in the sleep lab, your doctor may want you to take one or more daytime sleep tests as well.

One, called the multiple sleep latency test, measures how long it takes you to drift off while lying down in a quiet room and also determines what stages of sleep you experience during a brief nap. The procedure is usually repeated four or more times during the day at two-hour intervals. This test assesses how sleepy a person is and looks for signs of narcolepsy. Falling asleep within five minutes each time indicates extreme sleepiness. A person who enters REM sleep very quickly (within about 20 minutes) likely has narcolepsy.

In a less common test, called the maintenance of wakefulness test, you're given the opposite instructions: try to stay awake. This ability is also affected by the degree of sleepiness. People are sometimes given both tests at different times. One use of this test is by the Federal Aviation Association, which requires

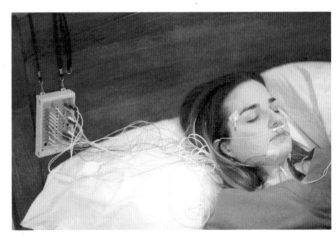

Polysomnography is commonly done in sleep labs. For this procedure, small electrodes placed on the scalp and other parts of the body take readings during the night. Lab staff examine the readings from a nearby control room.

pilots treated for sleep apnea to show that they are sufficiently awake and alert to fly.

Home-based tests

For people who, based on their symptoms, probably have moderate to severe obstructive sleep apnea and who have no other significant medical problems, home sleep monitoring may be almost as effective as a night in the sleep lab. Portable home recording devices also may be used when polysomnography is not available and a person's symptoms suggest a need for immediate treatment or when a person is bedridden or medically unstable and cannot be moved. Finally, home-based tests can provide an easy way for a physician to evaluate the effectiveness of a treatment.

The big advantage of a home sleep test is its convenience. You sleep in your own bed, not an unfamiliar hospital bed, and you do the test based on your schedule, not when a sleep center can fit you in. But there are disadvantages, too. There's no technician around to reattach a sensor or wire if it comes loose, so you must repeat the test if this happens. In addition, home monitors detect only OSA, not other sleep disorders, which means that some people still end up needing a full sleep lab test. And because home-based tests are not as sensitive, they may understate the severity of OSA or miss mild sleep apnea altogether. If home testing is appropriate for you, your doctor may loan you a kit or order one for you through one of the companies that have sprung up to provide this service.

Apnea detectors. Portable detection kits come in many makes and models. There are simple ones that measure only the amount of oxygen in the bloodstream. Most also monitor other breathing variables—air flow, chest movement (to detect breathing patterns), and heart rate or the heart's electrical activity. Some portable devices can also detect snoring or leg movement. Very few measure brain activity and stages of sleep, information that is needed to identify other types of sleep disorders.

Once you have the kit, you attach the various sensors to your body before going to bed: a clip on your fingertip tracks your heart rate and the amount of oxygen in the bloodstream; a sensor that loops over the ears and sits below the nose monitors airflow and snoring; an elastic band around the chest records breathing patterns. With everything in place, you go to sleep in your own bed. The information is stored on a data card that your doctor downloads and interprets.

Wrist actigraphy. A wristwatch-sized monitoring device that automatically records arm or leg movements can be used to track periods of sleep and wakefulness at night. Although it cannot determine the stage of sleep, it can help clarify ambiguous aspects of a sleep diary—such as entries reporting long hours of sleep but exhaustion the next day—or assess the effectiveness of medical treatment. The actigraphy device may reveal that brief awakenings during the night are unknowingly disturbing sleep. In some studies, wrist actigraphy was almost 90% accurate in determining whether a person was asleep. This type of monitoring is now included in many wearable fitness devices and smart watches.

Looking forward to a healthier future

We hope that this report has given you a solid understanding of the various sleep disturbances and the ways they can harm your health. But it's worth taking a moment to look at the flip side—the benefits of routinely getting a good night's rest. The encouraging news is that if you successfully conquer whatever is preventing you from sleeping soundly, you can derive many benefits—not only more refreshing sleep at night, but also better energy, productivity, and mental well-being during the day. After a few weeks of healthy sleep, some people report feeling like a "whole new person." While there are no guarantees that you can always get eight hours of uninterrupted sleep, with proper treatment, you can reasonably expect improvements in your overall quality of life. ♥

Resources

Organizations

American Academy of Sleep Medicine
2510 N. Frontage Road
Darien, IL 60561
630-737-9700
www.sleepeducation.com

Dedicated to the advancement of sleep medicine and related research, this organization also provides the public with information on sleep disorders as well as contact information for accredited sleep centers.

American Sleep Apnea Association
1717 Pennsylvania Ave. NW, Suite 1025
Washington, DC 20012
888-293-3650 (toll-free)
www.sleepapnea.org

This nonprofit organization provides information on sleep apnea via brochures, a newsletter, and videos. It also operates a network of support groups throughout the country.

Narcolepsy Network
46 Union Drive, #A212
North Kingston, RI 02852
888-292-6522 (toll-free)
www.narcolepsynetwork.org

This organization offers educational materials on narcolepsy, as well help in finding support groups.

National Center on Sleep Disorders Research
National Heart, Lung, and Blood Institute, NIH
6701 Rockledge Drive
Bethesda, MD 20892
301-435-0199
www.nhlbi.nih.gov/about/org/ncsdr

This federal center, part of the National Institutes of Health, coordinates government-supported sleep research, training, and education. It offers a number of free publications about sleep disorders.

National Sleep Foundation
1010 N. Glebe Road, Suite 310
Arlington, VA 22201
703-243-1697
www.sleepfoundation.org

This nonprofit foundation helps consumers locate sleep centers and provides information on a variety of sleep topics.

Restless Legs Syndrome Foundation, Inc.
3006 Bee Caves Road, Suite D206
Austin, TX 78746
512-366-9109
www.rls.org

This nonprofit foundation distributes brochures and provides information on restless legs syndrome. It also maintains a list of support groups located throughout the country.

Websites

Conquering Insomnia Program
www.cbtforinsomnia.com

This cognitive behavioral therapy program, developed at Harvard Medical School and the University of Massachusetts Medical Center, is available for purchase as either an online program or in CD format.

Sleep and Health Education Program
http://healthysleep.med.harvard.edu

Created by Harvard Medical School's Division of Sleep Medicine and the WGBH Educational Foundation, this site aims to help the general public understand sleep and to get the sleep they need.

Sleep Healthy Using the Internet
www.shuti.net

This interactive Web-based program, developed at the University of Virginia Center for Behavioral Medicine Research, provides cognitive behavioral therapy for insomnia.

Welltrinsic Sleep Network
www.welltrinsic.com

The website for this nationwide network of board-certified sleep specialists and accredited sleep centers includes a "Find a Sleep Doctor" feature.